Rad Tech's Guide to MRI

Rad Tech's Guide to MRI

Basic Physics, Instrumentation, and Quality Control

Second Edition

William H. Faulkner, Jr., B.S.,R.T.(R)(MR)
(CT), FSMRT, MRSO (MRSC™)
William Faulkner & Associates, LLC
Chattanooga, TN, USA

Series Editor

Euclid Seeram, PhD, FCAMRT

WILEY Blackwell

This edition first published 2020
© 2020 John Wiley & Sons Ltd

Edition History
Wiley-Blackwell (1e, 2001)

The right of William H. Faulkner, Jr. to be identified as the author of this work has been asserted in accordance with law.

Registered Office(s)
John Wiley & Sons, Inc., 111 River Street, Hoboken, NJ 07030, USA
John Wiley & Sons Ltd, The Atrium, Southern Gate, Chichester, West Sussex, PO19 8SQ, UK

Editorial Office
9600 Garsington Road, Oxford, OX4 2DQ, UK

For details of our global editorial offices, customer services, and more information about Wiley products visit us at www.wiley.com.

Wiley also publishes its books in a variety of electronic formats and by print-on-demand. Some content that appears in standard print versions of this book may not be available in other formats.

Limit of Liability/Disclaimer of Warranty

Library of Congress Cataloging-in-Publication Data

Names: Faulkner Jr., William H., author.
Title: Rad tech's guide to MRI : basic physics, instrumentation, and
   quality control / William H. Faulkner, Jr.
Other titles: Guide to MRI : basic physics, instrumentation, and quality
   control | Rad tech series.
Description: 2nd edition. | Hoboken, NJ : John Wiley & Sons Limited, 2020.
   | Series: Rad tech's guides | Includes index.
Identifiers: LCCN 2019040590 (print) | LCCN 2019040591 (ebook) | ISBN
   9781119508571 (paperback) | ISBN 9781119509486 (adobe pdf) | ISBN
   9781119509509 (epub)
Subjects: MESH: Magnetic Resonance Imaging–methods | Magnetic Resonance
   Imaging–instrumentation | Quality Control
Classification: LCC RC386.6.M34 (print) | LCC RC386.6.M34 (ebook) | NLM
   WN 185 | DDC 616.07/548–dc23
LC record available at https://lccn.loc.gov/2019040590
LC ebook record available at https://lccn.loc.gov/2019040591

Cover Design: Wiley
Cover Image: © Andrew Brookes / Getty Images

Set in 11.5/13.5pt STIX Two Text by SPi Global, Pondicherry, India

SKY10100564_032025

For Tricia, Amber and Zooey

Contents

1 Hardware Overview

Instrumentation: Magnets

To obtain a **magnetic resonance (MR) signal** from tissues, a large static magnetic field is required. The primary purpose of the static magnetic field (known as the B_0 field) is to magnetize the tissue. The magnet technology utilized is either referred to as: Permanent, Resistive or Superconductive. Regardless of the style or type of magnet used, the B_0 field must be stable and homogeneous, particularly in the central area of the magnet (isocenter) which is where the anatomy to be imaged should be placed.

- The vertical field magnet design uses two magnets, one above the patient and one below the patient.
- The frame, which supports the magnets, also serves to "return" the magnetic field.
- Generally, vertical magnets have a reduced fringe field compared with conventional horizontal field magnets.

Rad Tech's Guide to MRI: Basic Physics, Instrumentation, and Quality Control, Second Edition. William H. Faulkner, Jr.
© 2020 John Wiley & Sons Ltd. Published 2020 by John Wiley & Sons Ltd.

- The "open design" of these systems is often marketed as being less confining to the patient who may be anxious or claustrophobic.
- "Open MRI" is marketing terminology and has no basis or meaning in science.
- The radio-frequency (RF) transmit coil and gradient coils for vertical field magnets (discussed in more detail later) are flat coils located on the "face" of the magnets.
- The *receiver* or surface coils used with vertical field magnets are solenoid in design.
- For vertical field magnets, field strength and homogeneity can be increased by reducing the gap between the two magnets. The disadvantage to reducing the gap is the obvious reduction in patient area.

Regardless of whether the field is vertical or horizontal, there are three primary types of technology utilized tor MRI system magnets: permanent, resistive, and superconducting.

Permanent Magnets

- MRI systems based on permanent magnet technology use materials which are, as the name implies, permanently magnetized to produce the main external magnetic field (B_O).
- Increasing the amount of material used increases the field strength, in addition to size and weight.
- Permanent magnets generally have field strengths of 0.06 to 0.35 Tesla.
- Generally, vertical field permanent magnets have a relatively small fringe field.
- Because of the small fringe field, permanent magnets are often easy to sight, though their weight can be an issue.
- Permanent magnets are sensitive to ambient room temperature.
- Changes in scan room temperature can cause the field strength to vary several gauss per degree.

- Because changes in field strength result in changes in resonant frequency, image quality can vary if the field drifts significantly.

Resistive Magnets

- Resistive magnets are generally used in either a vertical or transverse field system.
- Larger resistive magnet-based systems can have field strengths up to 0.6 Tesla.
- Whenever electrical current is applied to a wire, a magnetic field is induced around the wire.
- To produce a static field (i.e. not alternating), direct current is required.
- Resistive systems generally also contain an iron core around which the wire is wound.
- Increasing the amount of current or turns of wire increases the field strength and results in heat in the wire.
- Resistive magnets require a constant current to maintain the static field.
- Cooling of the coils is also required as the by-product of electrical resistance is heat.
- Resistive magnets can easily be turned off when not in use (permanent and superconductive magnets cannot be turned off).
- The earliest type of magnets used in MRI were resistive.
- Resistive magnets can also be temperature-sensitive.

Superconductive Magnets

- Superconductive magnets are similar to resistive magnets because they use direct current actively applied to a coil of wire to produce the static magnetic field.
- The main difference is that the coils are immersed in liquid helium (cryogen) to remove the resistance.
- When the temperature of any conductor is reduced, electrical resistance decreases.

- Without the resistance, the electrical current can flow within a closed circuit without external power being applied (i.e. no voltage is needed for current to flow).
- The flow of electrical current without resistance is known as superconductivity.
- Most superconductive magnets are solenoid in design and thus, result in a horizontal magnetic field.
- Recent innovations in magnet design allow for vertical field systems using superconductive magnets.
- Superconductive magnets are capable of achieving higher field strengths compared to permanent and resistive magnet technology.
- Small-bore horizontal magnets used to image small animals and tissue samples can have field strengths of 10 Tesla or higher.
- Superconductive magnets currently approved for use by the FDA (US) in clinical settings include field strengths from 1.0 Tesla to 7.0 Tesla.
- Higher field strengths produce greater fringe fields.
- To reshape and/or reduce the fringe field for siting purposes, magnetic shielding is employed.
- Passive magnetic shielding uses metal (iron) in the scan room walls.
- Active magnetic shielding uses additional coils as part of the magnet design.
- Helium is not stable as a liquid. The temperature of liquid helium is 4 Kelvin. In order to maintain that temperature, it must be kept in a vacuum. Helium will boil at 4.2 K. If the temperature within the vessel containing the magnet coils and liquid helium rises only slightly, or if the vacuum were to be lost, then the liquid helium will boil and expand at a ratio of approximately 1:750.
- The resultant helium gas will burst through a pressure-sensitive containment system and should vent outside the scan room through a duct system attached to the magnet.

- In the absence of the supercooled environment, the current in the magnet coils will experience resistance, and the static field will be lost.
- This sudden and violent loss of superconductivity is referred to as a *quench*.
- The major advantage of superconducting technology is high field strength, which results in inherently high signal-to-noise ratio (SNR).
- The high SNR can be "traded" for rapid scan times and increased spatial resolution.
- The major disadvantage of superconducting technology is the high cost associated with acquisition, siting, and maintenance.

B_0 Homogeneity

Regardless of the type or style of magnet used for an MR system, the magnetic field must be as homogeneous as possible. This characteristic is particularly critical within the central area of the magnet (isocenter) where imaging takes place. The homogeneity is maximized through a process known as *shimming*. Shimming can be accomplished either *actively, passively,* or through a combination of both.

- Active shimming implies the use of additional coils within the magnet vessel or structure.
- Current applied in the shim coils either adds or subtracts from the static magnetic field to produce a field that is as homogeneous as possible.
- Passive shimming implies the use of small bits of ferrous material.
- In the case of a horizontal field magnet, the ferrous material is placed around the bore.
- In the case of a vertical field system, the material is placed on the face of the main magnets.

Instrumentation: RF Subsystem

Transmit

- The primary purpose of the RF subsystem is to transmit the RF pulses or RF field (known as the B1 field) and to receive the MR signal from tissue being examined.
- The B1 field is used to provide the necessary RF energy to cause the net magnetization of the tissues to tip and rotate through the transverse plane where the receiving coils are located.
- The RF subsystem consists of coils that transmit and/ or receive the RF signals and the electronics that power them.
- Most RF subsystems in use today are digital rather than analog.
- Digital RF systems provide for finer control of the RF pulses produced in the MRI process.
- RF coils can be designed to transmit only, receive only, or transmit and receive. The decision as to which design will be used is largely determined by the manufacturer or the overall MR system design.
- The most common type of RF receiving coils in use today are receive-only multichannel coils (sometimes referred to as "phased-array" coils).
- In superconductive, horizontal field systems, a large *body coil* is located within the magnet enclosure. In general, the body coil operates either as a transmit-only coil or as a transmit-and-receive (T/R) coil.
- Body coils are used to acquire information over a large field-of-view (FOV).
- The primary disadvantage of using the integrated body coil as a receive coil is an inherently low SNR.
- Generally, a larger coil will result in lower SNR. Conversely, a small coil will result in higher SNR.

- To increase the SNR, smaller surface (local) coils can be placed over or around the region of interest.
- Local coils can be either a T/R coil or a receive-only coil, again, largely based on the manufacturer's preference.
- If the local coil is a receive-only coil, then the integrated body coil transmits RF.
- Reducing the size of the local coil increases the SNR, but the area of coverage is reduced.

Local (Surface) Coils

The primary purpose of local coils is to increase the SNR. The main difficulty is to do so without excessive restriction of coverage of the area of interest. As mentioned, as the coil size is increased, the SNR is reduced. Currently, there are three main categories or types of local coils: linear, quadrature, and phased-array coils.

- The first type of local coils used in MRI were linear in design.
- Quadrature designs use additional loops and circuitry to improve the efficiency with which the MR signal is induced in the coil.
- Typically, quadrature coils produce an increase in the SNR of approximately 40% compared with a linear coil of the same size.
- Vertical field magnets require the use of solenoid coils because of the orientation of B_0. Generally, the solenoid configuration is more efficient compared with a liner coil of similar size.
- It is possible to combine coils electronically to improve signal uniformity through a region of interest.
- When two coils are combined in a manner such that they use the same receiver electronics, this is referred to as a *Helmholtz pair*.

- The Helmholtz pair has been used in coils designed to image the cervical spine, neck, and bilateral temporomandibular joints.
- Although a Helmholtz pair can improve the signal homogeneity across a region of interest, the SNR is not necessarily increased, which is primarily a result of coupling between the coils.
- Phased-array (multi-channel) coils allow for increased area of coverage without a reduction in the SNR.
- Typically, a phased-array coil consists of an array of coils designed to cover a particular area of the anatomy such as the spine, abdomen, or extremities.
- The major distinguishing characteristic of phased-array coil is that each active coil in the array is electronically connected to its own receiver.
- Multiple receivers can contribute to the increased coverage possible with a phased-array/multi-channel coil.
- With phased-array coils, one not only realizes the coverage of the entire array, but also the SNR characteristic of each coil within the array.
- RF coils must be "tuned" for the specific Larmor frequency of the MR system for which they are designed and cannot be used on systems operating at a different field strength.
- Generally, the tuning is set by the manufacturer and cannot be changed on site.

Instrumentation: Gradient Subsystem

The primary purpose of the gradient subsystem is to select the slice and imaging plane and to spatially encode the MR signal spatially. The gradient subsystem consists of gradient coils and the electronics that power them. The term gradient means slope or incline. A gradient magnetic field is, therefore, a magnet field that varies in intensity over distance. During the *imaging* process, gradient magnetic fields are also varied over time.

- Gradient magnetic fields are superimposed over the primary magnetic field.
- Gradient magnetic fields are produced as current is applied to the gradient coils.
- There are three sets of gradient coils in MR systems.
- The coil that is used to vary the intensity of the magnetic field in the head-to-foot direction is referred to as a *z gradient coil.*
- The coil that is used to vary the intensity of the magnetic field in the right-to-left direction is referred to as an *x gradient coil.*
- The coil that is used to vary the intensity of the magnetic field in the anterior-to-posterior direction is referred to as a *y gradient coil.*
- The term *amplitude* refers to the severity or steepness of the slope of the gradient magnetic field.
- A high-amplitude gradient will have a steep slope and will, therefore, greatly vary the intensity of the magnetic field in a given direction.
- *Polarity* (either positive or negative) refers to whether the gradient magnetic field is creating a field greater than or less than the frequency of B_0.
- The maximum amplitude of gradient magnetic fields is described in units of millitesla per meter (mT/m) or Tesla per meter (T/m).
- Higher gradient amplitudes offer the benefits of thinner slices and smaller FOVs.
- The speed at which a gradient magnetic field attains its maximum amplitude is identified by its *rise time.*
- Rise time is expressed in units of microseconds (μsec).
- Another way to express gradient performance is *slew rate.*

- Slew rate is defined as the maximum amplitude divided by the rise time.
- Slew rate is expressed in units of Tesla/meter/second (T/m/sec).
- Increased slew rates offer the benefit of reduced echo times (TE), increased number of slices per repetition time (TR), shorter TR for three-dimensional (3D) sequences, and improved image quality with echo planar and fast-spin-echo sequences.

2 Fundamental Principles

Electromagnetism: Faraday's Law of Induction

Electricity and magnetism go hand-in-hand. Whenever an electrical current is produced in a wire, a magnetic field is produced around the wire. As the current in the wire increases, the magnetic field increases. This characteristic is the basic principle behind the construction of resistive and superconductive magnets discussed in Chapter 1. Magnets or magnetic fields can also be used to induce electrical current in conductors. This principle is known as *Faraday's Law of Induction* and is written as $\Delta B/\Delta t = \Delta V$ Faraday's Law of Induction states that moving a magnet or changing a magnetic field (ΔB) over time (Δt) in the presence of a conductor will induce a voltage (ΔV) in the conductor. As the magnetic field moving through the conductor is increased, the current induced in the conductor is increased. As the time decreases (shortens) – in other words, the more rapid the change in the magnetic field – the more the induced current is increased. Faraday's Law of Induction is the basic principle by which MR signals are induced within the receiver coil.

Rad Tech's Guide to MRI: Basic Physics, Instrumentation, and Quality Control, Second Edition. William H. Faulkner, Jr.
© 2020 John Wiley & Sons Ltd. Published 2020 by John Wiley & Sons Ltd.

Magnetism

Magnetic Properties of Matter

All matter has magnetic properties. There are three types of magnetic properties: diamagnetic, paramagnetic, and ferromagnetic.

- Diamagnetic substances have paired electrons in their orbital shells.
- Diamagnetic substances exhibit a slight negative or repelling effect when placed in an externally applied magnetic field.
- Diamagnetic substances are said to have a −1 susceptibility.
- The diamagnetic effect is weak.
- Gold is an example of a diamagnetic substance.
- Paramagnetic substances have unpaired electrons in their orbital shells.
- Paramagnetic substances become magnetized when placed in an externally applied magnetic field.
- Paramagnetic substances do not retain magnetization when removed from an externally applied field.
- Paramagnetic substances are said to have a + 1 susceptibility.
- Gadolinium is an example of a paramagnetic substance.
- The paramagnetic properties of gadolinium are the reason it is used in contrast agents for magnetic resonance imaging (MRI).
- Some substances have both diamagnetic and paramagnetic properties. In this event, since the paramagnetic effects are stronger, the substance exhibits paramagnetic characteristics.
- Ferromagnetic substances are similar to paramagnetic substances in that they become magnetized when placed in an externally applied magnetic field.

▨ Ferromagnetic substances, however, will remain magnetized when the externally applied field is removed.
▨ Iron is an example of a ferromagnetic substance.
▨ A dipole is a magnet with two poles: north and south.
▨ By convention, the magnetic field of a dipole runs from the north pole around to the south pole.
▨ When two identical poles are brought together, the resultant fields oppose each other and thus they repel.
▨ When two opposite poles are brought together, the resultant fields combine and the two magnets are pulled toward each other.
▨ The strength of a magnetic field is expressed in terms of Gauss or Tesla.
▨ Gauss is the CGS (Centimeter-Gram-Second) unit of magnetic flux density.
▨ Tesla is the International Standard (SI) unit of magnetic flux density.
▨ The earth's magnetic field strength is approximately 0.5 G.
▨ One Tesla equals 10 000 G.

Nuclear Magnetism

In the early days of MRI, the term *nuclear magnetic resonance* (NMR) was used. The word *nuclear,* however, elicited visions of radioactivity, thus the name was changed to MRI. In reality, the term *nuclear* as it is used in NMR refers to the nucleus of atoms. Atoms which have an odd number of protons in their nucleus are "magnetically active." This means that certain nuclei have properties that cause them to display magnetic characteristics. Of all the magnetically active nuclei, hydrogen is the most abundant in the human body and is, therefore, the most commonly used in clinical MRI.

▨ The hydrogen atom consists of a single proton.
▨ The proton has mass, a positive charge, and spins on its axis.

- The spinning motion of a positively charged particle results in a magnetic field around the proton.
- The proton's magnetic field is often termed the *magnetic moment.*
- For this reason, hydrogen is considered *magnetically active.*
- Other nuclei (e.g. carbon, phosphorus, sodium) are also magnetically active because of their nuclear makeup.
- Hydrogen, however, is nearly 100% abundant in the human body and has a relatively large magnetic moment.
- In the human body, water and fat are the most abundant molecules with hydrogen.
- For these reasons, hydrogen is ideal for use in MRI.

Behavior of Hydrogen in a Magnetic Field

Because the hydrogen proton, or *spin,* has a magnetic moment, it exhibits certain behavior when placed in a large, externally applied magnetic field (B_0).

Alignment and Net Magnetization

- Within seconds of tissue being placed in a magnetic field, the hydrogen protons will assume one of two possible spin states or energy levels: high-energy or low-energy.
- One way to explain or visualize the spin states is to refer to the protons as aligning with or against the external magnetic field.
- Spins aligned parallel (i.e. with the direction of B_0) are said to be in the low-energy state.
- Spins aligned antiparallel (i.e. against the direction of B_0) are said to be in the high-energy state.

- After several seconds of placing tissue in an externally applied magnetic field, there will be a slight majority of spins in the low-energy state (parallel).
- The magnetic moments of spins in the high-energy state cancel the effect of an equal number of spins in the low-energy state.
- Since there is a slightly greater number of spins in the low-energy state compared with the high-energy state, the magnetic moments of these spins, in the so-called *spin excess,* add to form the magnetic field of the tissue and that is referred to as the *net magnetization vector* (NMV).
- The NMV is therefore aligned parallel to B_0 (external static magnetic field).
- This condition, as just described, reached within a few seconds of placing tissues in an external field is known as *thermal equilibrium.*
- The energy delta (or difference) between the two spin states is field-strength dependent.
- As B0 is increased, the energy delta between the two spin states will increase.
- Though there is always a greater number of spins aligned parallel versus antiparallel at higher field strengths, there is a greater number when compared with lower field strengths.
- For this reason, the tissue magnetization (i.e. NMV) is greater at higher field strengths.

Precession

- The hydrogen protons also precess around the axis of the static magnetic field.
- The precession motion of the proton is often compared with the motion of a spinning top or gyroscope.
- The spinning gyroscope exerts a force (spin angular momentum) perpendicular to the direction of the spin.

- Gravity pulls downward causing the gyroscope to wobble or precess.
- With the hydrogen proton, the spinning motion of the proton produces spin angular momentum in the same fashion.
- Additionally, the proton exhibits a magnetic field (magnetic moment).
- The ratio of the spins angular momentum to its magnetic moment is known as the *gyromagnetic ratio.*
- The gyromagnetic ratio varies with each magnetically active nucleus and is expressed in units of megahertz/Tesla (MHz/T).
- The gyromagnetic ratio for hydrogen is 42.58 MHz/T.
- The actual precessional frequency for hydrogen can be calculated from the Larmor equation (Figure 2.1).
- Increasing B_0 causes the precessional or resonant frequency of hydrogen to increase. Decreasing B_0 causes the resonant frequency to decrease.
- The frequency at which the hydrogen protons precess is known as the *Larmor frequency* or *resonant frequency.*

$$\omega_0 = B_0 \cdot \gamma$$

1.5 T × 42.6 MHz/T = 63.9 MHz

3.0 T × 42.6 MHz/T = 127.8 MHz

Figure 2.1 The effect of field strength on the precessional frequency is shown. As the field strength increases, the processional frequency increases.

A little more about thermal equilibrium:

- At thermal equilibrium, the hydrogen spins do not precess at exactly the same frequency.
- Several factors contribute to their lack of phase coherence. Primarily, hydrogen spins are inhomogeneities and chemical shift effects.
- Inhomogeneities in the magnetic field are always present. Although the magnet is *shimmed,* when a patient is placed in the magnet, the field is distorted.

- Inhomogeneities also occur within the body, which are known as *local field inhomogeneities.*
- Local inhomogeneities can be caused by metal or foreign materials in the body, as well as by areas with vastly different magnetic properties.
- When metal is present within the body, the magnetic field around the metal is greatly distorted.
- This distortion causes the resonant frequencies of the spins to vary greatly.
- Smaller distortions are observed at air-tissue interfaces. Although these distortions cause a variance in the spin's resonant frequencies, the amount of variance (i.e. dephasing) is not as great when compared with the presence of metal objects or implants.
- The molecular environment can also affect the phase coherence among the spins.
- A water molecule consists of oxygen and hydrogen. The oxygen atom "steals" the hydrogen's electron. As a result, the hydrogen proton "experiences" the external magnetic field without the normal presence of its orbital electron.
- A fat molecule consists of carbon and hydrogen. The carbon atom does not alter the orbit of the hydrogen's electron. As a result, the hydrogen proton "experiences" the external field with its orbital electron in place.
- The absence of the orbital electron causes the proton in a water molecule to experience a slightly higher field than the proton in a fat molecule.
- Hydrogen in water will therefore precess slightly faster than hydrogen in fat.
- This difference in precessional frequency is known as *chemical shift.*
- The amount of chemical shift (i.e. frequency difference) is field-strength dependent.
- However, chemical shift, when expressed independently of field strength, is expressed as 3.5 parts per million (ppm).

- The amount of chemical shift in units of Hertz depends on the field strength.
- For example, at 1.5 Tesla, 1 ppm = 63.86 Hz. Therefore 3.5 ppm = 224 Hz, which means that hydrogen in water will precess 224 Hz faster than the hydrogen in fat.
- The effect of local field inhomogeneities and chemical shift causes the spins to precess out of phase at thermal equilibrium.

3 Production of Magnetic Resonance Signal

he magnetic resonance (MR) signal is induced in a receiver coil when the net magnetization vector (NMV) is rotated through the coil. This chapter will examine how this process is accomplished. When describing this process, a 3D Cartesian graph will be utilized. The vertical (or z) direction will indicate the direction of the external field (B_0). Magnetization aligned in this direction will be referred to as *Mz* or *longitudinal magnetization*. Magnetization in the perpendicular axis or plane (*x, y*) will be referred to as *Mxy* or *transverse magnetization*.

- Radio-frequency (RF) energy at the frequencies utilized in MRI is nonionizing, electromagnetic radiation.
- A radio wave consists of oscillating magnetic and electric fields.
- Exposing magnetized tissue to an RF field at the Larmor frequency (dictated by the strength of B_0), first causes the hydrogen spins to begin precessing *in phase*, which causes the NMV to precess as well.
- As the application of the RF continues, some of the spins in the low-energy state absorb energy from the RF field and move to the high-energy state.

Rad Tech's Guide to MRI: Basic Physics, Instrumentation, and Quality Control, Second Edition. William H. Faulkner, Jr.
© 2020 John Wiley & Sons Ltd. Published 2020 by John Wiley & Sons Ltd.

- As more and more spins absorb energy, changing spin states, the NMV begins to tip outward, away from the longitudinal or z axis.
- When the spins are evenly distributed between the two spin states, the NMV will now be precessing through the x, y (transverse) plane, 90° away from its original orientation in the z axis (Figure 3.1).
- Tipping the NMV 90° away from the z axis is referred to as applying a 90° flip angle.
- Another way to phrase the effects of applying a 90° flip angle is to say that the longitudinal magnetization (Mz) is converted to transverse magnetization (Mxy).

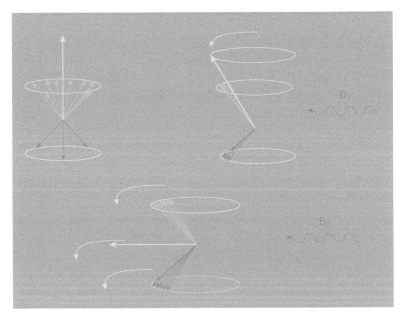

Figure 3.1 The effect of applying a radio-frequency (RF) pulse at the resonant or Larmor frequency is demonstrated. (a) The spins begin to precess in phase. As a result, the NMV also precesses. (b) As the pulse continues, some of the spins in the low-energy state gain energy from the RF pulse and move to the high-energy state, which causes NMV to tip outward and to precess through the transverse (xy) plane.

- Increasing the amount of RF energy will cause an increase in the flip angle.
- To double the flip angle, a fourfold increase in RF power is required.
- The amount of power necessary to achieve a desired flip angle will depend on several factors, including the field strength and the type of RF coil used for transmitting the RF signal and is determined during *prescan* or the "tuning" phase performed before each scan.
- When the desired flip angle is achieved, the RF pulse is discontinued to allow for detection of the signal.
- As the NMV is precessing through the xy plane, it will precess through a receiver coil oriented in the same plane (Figure 3.2).
- In accordance with Faraday's Law of Induction, an MR signal will be induced in the coil.

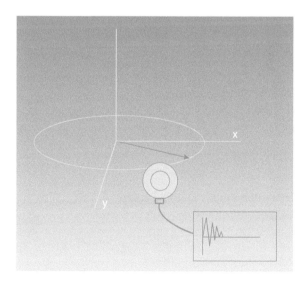

Figure 3.2 As the NMV is precessing through the xy plane, it will precess through a receiver coil, which is oriented in the same plane.

- The signal induced in a receiver coil immediately following an RF excitation pulse is known as the *free induction decay* (FID).
- The FID decays rapidly after removal of the RF pulse (see Figure 3.2).
- The FID is a result of the shrinking of the tissues' transverse magnetization as it rotates through the xy plane.
- The NMV shrinks because spins rapidly lose phase coherence after the RF pulse has been removed.
- Simultaneously but independently, some of the spins in the high-energy state lose energy gained from the RF pulse and return to the low-energy state.
- As more spins return to the low-energy state, the NMV again increases in z or longitudinal direction.

4 Relaxation and Tissue Characteristics

Following excitation by the radio-frequency (RF) pulse, the spins (hydrogen protons) undergo relaxation returning to thermal equilibrium. Relaxation consists of two simultaneous yet independent processes; T1 and T2-relaxation.

T2-Relaxation

- T2-relaxation is also referred to as *"Spin-Spin."*
- It occurs due to an *exchange of energy* between the spins (hydrogen protons).
- T2-relaxation results in a *decay of transverse magnetization.*
- T1-relaxation is also referred to as *"Spin-lattice."*
- It occurs due to a *loss of energy* from the spins (hydrogen protons) to their *molecular lattice.*
- T1-relaxation results in a *recovery of longitudinal magnetization.*
- Both T2-relaxation and T1-relaxation rates are *exponential.*
- The T2-relaxation time of a tissue is defined as when *63% of transverse magnetization has decayed.*

Rad Tech's Guide to MRI: Basic Physics, Instrumentation, and Quality Control, Second Edition. William H. Faulkner, Jr.
© 2020 John Wiley & Sons Ltd. Published 2020 by John Wiley & Sons Ltd.

- Water is a small molecule and, as such, exhibits a rapid molecular tumbling rate. The rapid molecular tumbling rate results in a relatively long T2-relaxation time.
- Fat is a much larger molecule and, as such, exhibits a slower molecular tumbling rate. This results in fat having a relatively short T2-relaxation time.
- T2-relaxation times are only slightly affected by field strength (not clinically significant).
- The temperature of the tissue when sampled will affect the molecular tumbling rate and, as such, will affect the T2-relaxation time.

T1-Relaxation

- The T1-relaxation time of a tissue is defined as when *63% of longitudinal magnetization has recovered.*
- Water (due to its size and therefore molecular tumbling rate) has a relatively long T1-relaxation time compared to fat (short T1-relaxation time).
- T1-relaxation times of tissue vary significantly with field strength.
- Increasing the field strength lengthens the T1-relaxation time of tissues.
- The temperature of the tissue when sampled will affect the molecular tumbling rate and, as such, will affect the T1-relaxation time of the tissue.
- **It is not necessary to memorize actual T1- and T2-relaxation times of tissue as they will vary depending on the conditions under which they are sampled (field strength and temperature).**

Proton Density

- Proton density is a measure of proton concentration in a given volume of tissue (basically a "head-count" of hydrogen protons).

- Tissues with higher proton density will have greater inherent Magnetic Resonance (MR) signal.
- Proton density is therefore a major factor in MR signal strength in Magnetic Resonance Imaging (MRI).
- Pure cerebro-spinal fluid (CSF) has the highest proton density of all normal occurring substances in the human body.
- Proton density is expressed as a percentage relative to CSF.
- *CSF has a proton density of 100%.*

T2* (Pronounced "T2 star")

- Following an RF pulse, the transverse magnetization decays as the spins (protons) lose phase coherence.
- One reason for loss of phase coherence is spin–spin interaction (or T2-relaxation).
- Another reason is *off-resonance effects.*
- Off-resonance effects result in dephasing due to *inhomogeneities in the static and local magnetic field and chemical shift* (resonant frequency differences between water and fat protons).
- The off-resonance effects are sometimes referred to as *T2' (pronounced "T2 prime").*
- The signal induced in a coil immediately following an RF pulse is referred to as the *Free Induction Decay* FID.
- The FID decay is therefore related to T2*.

5 Data Acquisition and Image Formation

Pulse Sequences

A pulse sequence, as the name implies, is a series of radio-frequency (RF) pulses. Control of the image contrast is accomplished by controlling the timing of the RF pulses in the pulse sequence, as well as by selecting the type of pulse sequence. The two primary types of pulse sequence are spin echo and gradient echo.

Spin Echo

- A spin echo pulse sequence begins with a 90° RF pulse followed by a 180° RF pulse.
- As previously discussed, the purpose of the 90° pulse is to convert the longitudinal magnetization to transverse magnetization.
- After the RF pulse is removed, the spins begin to rapidly dephase at a rate that is dependent on T2* free induction decay [FID].
- After a specified time, a 180° RF pulse is applied (Figure 5.1).

Rad Tech's Guide to MRI: Basic Physics, Instrumentation, and Quality Control, Second Edition. William H. Faulkner, Jr.
© 2020 John Wiley & Sons Ltd. Published 2020 by John Wiley & Sons Ltd.

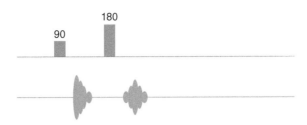

Figure 5.1 A simplified spin echo pulse sequence diagram (PSD).

- The purpose of the 180° RF pulse is to "flip" the magnetization through the transverse plane and refocus the spins that have dephased as a result of slight field inhomogeneities and chemical shifts (off-resonance effects).
- Any dephasing due to T2-relaxation is not affected or corrected for by the 180° RF pulse.
- As the spins refocus, or rephase, the magnetic resonance (MR) signal increases but then decreases once again as the spins dephase in the other "direction."
- The classic analogy is that of runners in a race. As the race begins, the faster runners get in front of the slower runners. If, at a specified point, the runners were to turn 180°, the faster runners will be behind the slower runners. As they return toward the starting line, the faster runners will catch the slower runners and they will all be *in phase* as they meet. As they continue, however, the faster runners will once again get ahead of the slower runners.
- In an MR pulse sequence, the operator can choose the time between the 90° pulse and the center of the echo. This parameter is known as the time to the echo (TE), usually expressed in milli-seconds (msec).
- One millisecond is equal to 1/1000 of a second.
- The 180° RF pulse is applied at a time equal to one half of the TE selected by the operator. For example, if the

operator selects a 20 msec TE, the 180° pulse will be automatically applied 10 msec after the 90° pulse.

- Occasionally, the time between the 90° pulse and the 180° pulse is referred to as ***tau***.
- This sequence (90–180) is repeated after a specified interval selected by the operator. This interval is known as the repetition time (TR).

Gradient Echo

- A gradient echo sequence begins with an RF pulse that may be 90° but can be greater or less than 90° when selected by the operator. This flip angle is selected based on the image contrast desired and will be discussed in more detail later.
- The initial (excitation) pulse in a gradient echo sequence may often be referred to as an *"Alpha pulse."*
- The echo is formed by the application of two gradient magnetic fields. The first gradient application dephases the spins (referred to as the *"dephasing lobe."* The second application of the gradient is the opposite polarity to the dephasing lobe, producing the exact opposite magnetic field (referred to as the *"rephasing lobe"*).
- The duration of the rephasing lobe is twice the duration of the dephasing lobe.
- Spins that sensed a reduction in the magnetic field and "slowed down" then sense an increase in the magnetic field and "speed up," refocusing the available transverse magnetization and producing an echo (Figure 5.2).
- As with the spin echo pulse sequence, the time between the initial or excitation pulse of the sequence and the center of the echo is the TE.
- The time between repetitions of the sequence is the TR.

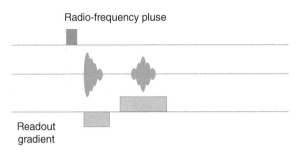

Figure 5.2 A simplified gradient echo pulse sequence diagram (PSD).

Inversion Recovery

When desired, a sequence can begin with a 180° inversion pulse. When done in a spin echo sequence, it is referred to as *inversion recovery*. An inversion pulse can be used with either a spin echo or gradient echo sequence. The time between the 180° inversion pulse and the 90° pulse in a spin echo sequence or the initial RF pulse in a gradient echo sequence is controlled by the operator and is known as the *time of inversion* or T1 (Figure 5.3).

Image Contrast Control

One of the major advantages of magnetic resonance imaging (MRI) over other types of imaging modalities is the ability to control the image contrast. Contrast observed on an MR image

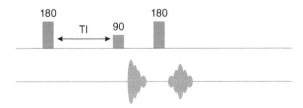

Figure 5.3 The time between the 180° inversion pulse and the 90° pulse in a spin echo sequence or the initial radio-frequency pulse in a gradient echo sequence is under operator control and is known as the time of inversion (TI).

depends on the intrinsic properties of tissues which include proton density (PD), T1- and T2-relaxation times, as well as the extrinsic parameters under the operator's control: TR, TE, time of inversion (TI), and flip angle. Unless specifically stated, the following refers to spin echo sequences only.

Time to the Echo and T2-Weighting

- As mentioned, in a spin echo sequence, the TE is the time between the initial 90° pulse and the center of the echo.
- Because the 180° pulse does not correct for any loss of dephasing from spin–spin or T2 relaxation, the quicker the echo is formed, the less the loss of magnetization (and therefore loss of signal) due to T2 relaxation.
- Acquiring a sequence with a longer TE will increase the amount of T2 decay that occurs between the 90° pulse and the echo.
- An image acquired with an extremely short TE (e.g. 20 msec or less) will therefore have fewer effects from T2 decay (as opposed to a longer TE).
- An image acquired with a longer TE (e.g. 80 msec or higher) will therefore exhibit a greater amount of contrast from the T2 differences between tissues.
- In this way, TE controls the amount of T2 contrast in an MR image. Reducing the TE reduces the T2 weighting in the image. Increasing the TE increases the T2 weighting in the image (Figure 5.4).

Repetition Time and T1-Weighting

- As mentioned, the TR is the time between repetitions of the pulse sequence.
- The longer the TR selected, the greater the amount of time allowing for regrowth of the longitudinal magnetization (Mz) between repetitions of the pulse sequence.

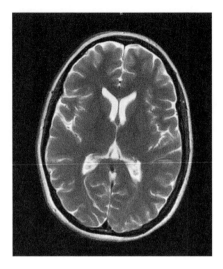

Figure 5.4 T2-weighted image.

- When a short TR is selected (e.g. 400 msec), only the spins with a short T1 time (such as fat) will be given sufficient time to recover and, as such, will exhibit a higher signal. Spins with longer T1 times (such as water or cerebrospinal fluid [CSF]) will be more saturated (i.e. they will exhibit less longitudinal recovery) and, as such, will exhibit a lower signal
- If a longer TR is selected (e.g. 3000 msec), all spins will be given more time for longitudinal recovery to occur.
- In this way, TR controls the amount of T1 contrast in an MR image. Reducing the TR increases the T1 weighting in the image. Increasing the TR reduces the T1 weighting in the image (Figure 5.5).

Combining Repetition Time and Time to the Echo to Control Image Contrast

If an image with T1 weighting is desired, then a short TE is selected (20 msec or less). Using a short TE does not make an image T1-weighted, but rather, it makes it less T2-weighted.

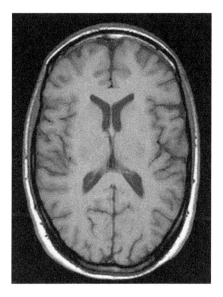

Figure 5.5 T1-weighted image.

Selecting a short TR (approximately 400–700 msec) will then produce an image with T1 weighting. The exact TR depends on the tissues being imaged and the field strength (because T1 times are field-strength dependent).

If an image with T2 weighting is desired, then a long TR is selected (3000 msec or higher). Using a long TR does not make an image T2-weighted, but rather, it makes it less T1-weighted. Selecting a long TE (80 msec or higher) will then produce an image with T2 weighting. Increasing the TR from 3000 msec will increase the signal from CSF or water and will therefore increase the contrast between certain structures. As a general rule, in the brain and spine, TR times of 4000 msec or higher will produce images with high contrast between CSF and surrounding structures.

If PD weighting is desired, a short TE is selected (20 msec or less) to reduce the T2 weighting. A long TR is then selected (3500 msec or higher) to reduce the T1 weighting (Figure 5.6).

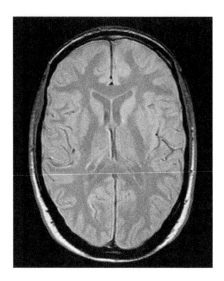

Figure 5.6 Proton density-weighted image.

When acquiring PD-weighted images in the brain, generally, a TR of between 2000 and 3000 msec is selected. As mentioned, when higher TR times are selected, the signal intensity from CSF is increased. A high signal from CSF may actually reduce the contrast between certain abnormalities and CSF. Multiple sclerosis (MS) plaques are a good example. MS plaques usually occur in the periventricular white matter and have a moderately high signal on PD-weighted images. If the signal intensity from CSF is too high, then the plaques may be indistinguishable from the adjacent CSF. In any event, increasing the TR will increase the signal intensity from CSF and vice versa.

Gradient Echo Contrast Control

Using gradient echo sequences, images with T-2 or PD-contrasts (i.e. bright fluid) can be acquired using short TR times. The benefit of this technique is a reduction in scanning times over sequences using longer TR times. Up to this point, we have been assuming that the pulse sequence begins with a 90° pulse. In gradient echo sequences, the flip angle must be selected, as well as the TR and TE.

- If a short TR time is selected, then only the spins with short or rapid T1 times will be given sufficient time to recover longitudinal magnetization.
- To enable longitudinal recovery to occur with spins exhibiting long T1 times, lower flip angles are selected.
- As the flip angle is reduced (assuming constant TR), spins with longer T1 times exhibit greater longitudinal recovery and the image becomes less T1-weighted.
- In this way, flip angle controls T1.
- Reducing the flip angle has the same effect on image contrast as increasing the TR (i.e. the image becomes less T1-weighted).
- Increasing the flip angle has the same effect on image contrast as reducing the TR (i.e. the image becomes more T1-weighted).

Gradient Echo Sequences and T2*

As mentioned, the purpose of the 180° refocusing pulse in a spin echo pulse sequence is to refocus or correct for dephasing resulting from slight inhomogeneities and chemical shifts. In a gradient echo pulse sequence, the echo is formed by the reversal of a gradient magnetic field only (i.e. a 180° pulse is not used). Gradient echo sequences are often referred to as a gradient recalled echo (GRE) sequence. Because of the lack of the 180° RF pulse in a GRE sequence, the decay of transverse magnetization is a result of not only T2, but also the effects of local inhomogeneities and chemical shift. The addition of these off-resonance effects produces a more rapid rate of transverse magnetization decay, known as T2* (rather than T2) (Figure 5.7). *Steady State versus Spoiled.* The selection of a steady-state or spoiled sequence is based on the type of contrast desired (Figure 5.8).

$$\frac{1}{T2} + \frac{1}{T2'} = \frac{1}{T2*}$$

Figure 5.7 T2 represents spin–spin relaxation, T2′ represents the effects from inhomogeneities and chemical shift.

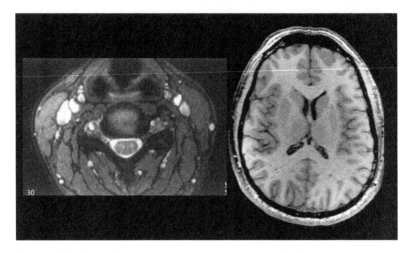

Figure 5.8 The axial cervical spine image on the left was acquired using a steady-state gradient recalled echo (GRE) sequence. The axial image of the brain on the right was acquired using a spoiled GRE sequence.

- When the TR is shorter than the T1 and T2* of tissues (generally less than 250 msec), a condition known as a *"steady state"* exists.
- In a steady state, longitudinal and transverse magnetization coexist as residual transverse magnetization exists from one TR to the next, because the short TR time does not allow for the normal transverse decay.
- Typically, when a steady-state GRE sequence is used, the signal from CSF remains bright regardless of the flip angle selected.
- This type of sequence may also be referred to as a *"coherent steady state."*

- To obtain T1-weighted images without the effects of the steady state (e.g. bright signal from fluid), a spoiled GRE sequence is used.
- The term *spoiling* refers to the removal of the residual transverse magnetization from the previous excitation pulse.
- Spoiling can be achieved by the use of a gradient magnetic field (gradient spoiling) or by varying the phase angle of the excitation pulse (RF spoiling).
- Images with heavy T1 weighting can be obtained with spoiled GRE sequences.
- Generally, when images with a high signal from fluid are desired (e.g. T2*- or PD-weighting), a steady state sequence is selected.
- When images with T1 contrast are desired, a spoiled sequence is selected.
- Spoiled GRE sequences are utilized when rapid T1-weighted images are desired following the administration of a Gadolinium-based MR contrast agent (e.g. liver, contrast-enhanced MRA, breast, etc.)

Balanced Gradient Echo

- A balanced gradient echo sequence is acquired such that the images' contrast is weighted for the difference between a tissue's T1- and T2-relaxation time (Figure 5.9).
- Tissues or substances which have a small difference between their T1- and T2-relaxation times are relatively low in signal.
- Tissues or substances which have a great difference between their T1- and T2-relaxation times will exhibit a high signal.
- Blood and fluid are two examples of tissues/substances with a high T1/T2 ratio or difference.
- Balanced GRE sequences have extremely short TR and TE times (the TE is always one half of the TR). As such, they are useful in cardiac MRI.

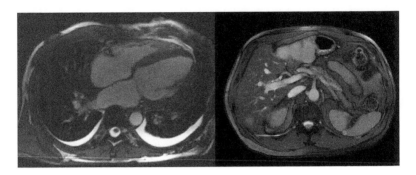

Figure 5.9 Balanced gradient recalled echo (GRE) images. Note the high signal from blood and fluid.

Inversion Recovery Contrast

Inversion recovery (IR) sequences were initially used to acquire images with strong T1 weighting. Although this application is still valid, newer rapid acquisition techniques (specifically Fast/Turbo Spin Echo) have emerged to allow for improved tissue contrasts and reduced scan times. Generally, inversion sequences begin with a 180° RF pulse to invert longitudinal magnetization (Mz). After the inversion, there is an operator-selectable delay time known as the TI. The TI time period may also be labeled as *"tau."* In a spin echo inversion sequence, the initializing 180° RF pulse (inversion pulse) is followed by a 90° pulse and then a 180° refocusing pulse. Inversion pulses may be available with other types of pulse sequences (e.g. GRE and/or echo planar imaging sequences). For the purposes of the following discussion, a spin echo inversion recovery sequence will be assumed.

- Following the application of the inversion pulse, the longitudinal magnetization will regrow along the z axis.
- If the 90° pulse is applied when a given tissue's magnetization has regrown to the zero or null point (i.e. neither negative nor positive), then the signal from the tissue will be null.

- As a rule, when a TI is selected that is 69% of a tissue's T1 time, the signal from the tissue will be zero (assuming a TR of sufficient length to allow for full longitudinal recovery).
- Therefore, the TI is selected based on the desired tissue contrast (i.e. the tissue or substance to be nulled.
- An inversion sequence that uses a short TI such that fat is nulled is often referred to as STIR (Short TI Recovery, or Short Tau Inversion Recovery).
- STIR sequences are often used in musculoskeletal examinations. In the presence of bone marrow diseases, normal bone marrow, which has a high fat content, will appear as a hypointense (dark) signal relative to lesions, which often have a high fluid content (Figure 5.10).
- In the brain, most diseased tissues are associated with an increase in fluid (edema).
- Using the standard, long TR and long TE spin echo sequence, it is often difficult to separate the high signal from pathologic fluid from the signal of CSF.

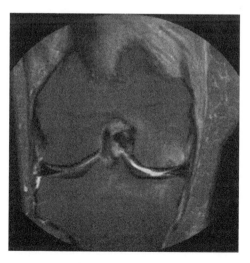

Figure 5.10 A Short tau inversion recovery (STIR) sequence with a time of inversion (TI) selected to null the signal from fat.

- With a Fluid Attenuated Inversion Recovery (FLAIR) sequence the TI is selected to null the signal from CSF.
- If a T2-weighted FLAIR is desired, a long TR (typically 8000 or greater) is selected as well as a long TE.
- The T1 and T2 times of pathologic fluid differ from the signal of CSF.
- For this reason, a diseased tissue exhibits a high signal (hyperintense) and CSF exhibits no signal when acquired using a T2-FLAIR sequence.
- T2-FLAIR sequences are useful for demonstrating strokes, infections, and white matter disease (Figure 5.11).
- An additional application of inversion sequences is to provide heavy T1 weighting.
- A relatively short TR (1800 to 2000 msec at 1.5 Tesla) is used along with a short TE (≤20 msec). The T1 is selected

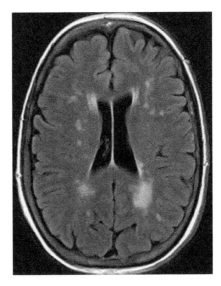

Figure 5.11 A T2-weighted fluid attenuated inversion recovery (T2-FLAIR) sequence, with a time of inversion (TI) selected to null the signal from cerebrospinal fluid (CSF).

once again to null the signal from CSF ($\cong 750$ msec at 1.5 Tesla).

- These sequences are useful in pediatric brain examinations. Because white matter is not fully myelinated until five years of age, it is difficult to obtain images with good gray-white contrast, particularly with a conventional spin echo sequence. Inversion sequences can provide excellent T1 weighting (Figure 5.12).

In summary, IR sequences provide an excellent tool for optimizing contrast. In the musculoskeletal system, STIR sequences suppress the normal marrow accentuating pathologic fluid. Although STIR sequences suppress or null the signal from fat, it is not specific to fat, and therefore it should not be used in conjunction with gadolinium. Gadolinium shortens the T1 time of water-based hydrogen protons almost to the T1 time of fat. STIR sequences can suppress the signal from gadolinium thus suppressing "enhancing" lesions. In brain examinations,

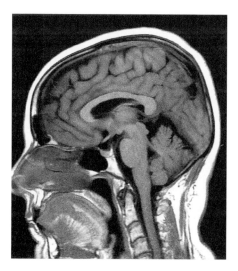

Figure 5.12 A T1-weighted inversion recovery sequence, which may be referred to as T1 FLAIR.

T2-FLAIR sequences improve visualization of pathology at CSF interfaces. Inversion sequences can also be used to provide heavily T1-weighted images of the brain. Whatever type of inversion sequence selected, it is important to remember that because T1 times are field-strength dependent, the TI required to null a particular tissue is also field-strength dependent. As field strength decreases, the appropriate TI decreases.

Image Formation

During the MR acquisition, data is collected when the echo is sampled. The data collected during the sampling of the echo (also known as *readout*) is digitized and mapped in relation to the spatial encoding gradients (phase and frequency). This mathematical map is referred to as *k-space*. One direction in k-space represents phase information and the other direction represents frequency information (Figure 5.13).

Physicists often use the letter *k* when referring to frequency. The number of data points in k-space is determined by the number of phase and frequency encodings selected by the operator. The

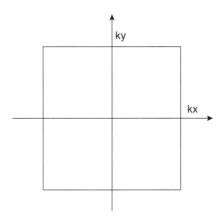

Figure 5.13 **K-space.** One direction in k-space represents phase information, whereas the other represents frequency.

central data points in k-space represent the low frequency data and contribute to the resultant images contrast and signal. The high-frequency data points in k-space contribute to the edge detail in the resultant image. The more high-frequency data collected during the acquisition, the greater the edge detail in the resultant image and, in some cases, the longer the scan time. Sampling all the data more than once results in reduced noise. When all the data points have been collected, the MR raw data (k-space data) is sent to the computer, and the image is reconstructed by a mathematical process known as *Fourier transform*. It is important to remember that k-space or raw data does not represent the MR image, but rather the data signal information as it relates to the gradient magnetic fields applied during the acquisition process.

The MR images overall "quality" is a function of image contrast, spatial resolution (edge detail) and the signal-to-noise ratio (SNR) in the acquired voxel. Image contrast is determined by the pulse sequence type and its associated parameters (e.g. TR, TE, TI, flip angle), as well as the tissue's PD and T1- and T2-(T2*) relaxation times. In this section, we will discuss how the other two characteristics (signal-to-noise and spatial resolution) are determined.

Data Acquisition

Three main functions are performed during a 2D data acquisition: slice selection, phase encoding, and frequency encoding (readout). As mentioned, there are three gradient coils inherent in our system. The purpose of the gradient coils is to produce a magnetic field that varies in intensity along a given direction and with time.

Physical Notation

- The gradient coil windings oriented to vary the magnetic field in the head-to-foot direction (regardless of the magnetic field orientation) is known as the z gradient coil.

The gradient coil windings oriented to vary the magnetic field in the right-to-left direction is known as the *x* gradient coil.

The gradient coil windings oriented to vary the magnetic field in the anterior-to-posterior direction is known as the *y* gradient coil.

As mentioned, three primary functions are required for MR data collection: slice selection, phase encoding, and frequency encoding. The three gradient coils are capable of performing any of the required functions depending on the choices made by the operator. Generally, when referring to the gradients by function rather than direction or orientation, the logical notation is used.

Logical Notation

The gradient used to perform slice selection is referred to as the *z* gradient.

The gradient used to perform phase encoding is referred to as the *y* gradient.

The gradient used to perform frequency encoding (readout) is referred to as the *x* gradient.

A good way to remember the logical notation is to place them in a logical order or alphabetically (x, y, and z). The functions can then be placed in alphabetical order with the corresponding gradient (frequency, phase, and slice).

When referring to a physical gradient or gradient magnetic field direction, the physical notation is used (Table 5.1).

When referring to a particular function of the gradients, the logical notation is used (see Table 5.1).

A simplified pulse sequence diagram (PSD) of a gradient echo sequence demonstrates the application of the gradients

Table 5.1 Physical and logical notations summary.

Physical Notation	Logical Notation	Gradient
Head/foot	Slice selection	z
Right/left	Frequency encoding	x
Anterior/posterior	Phase encoding	y

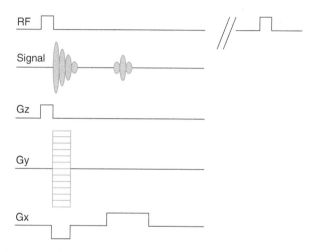

Figure 5.14 A pulse sequence diagram (PSD) shows the timing of the three major gradients: Gz = slice selection; Gy = phase encoding; Gx = frequency encoding (readout).

in relation to each other over time, labeled by their function (Figure 5.14). When referring to the function of the gradients in relation to a PSD, it is important to remember that the logical notation is used.

Slice Selection (2D)

- The first gradient to be applied is the slice selection gradient (z).
- The slice selection gradient is "on" during the application of the radio-frequency (RF) pulse. In a spin echo

sequence, the slice selection gradient is applied during both the 90° RF pulse and the 180° RF pulse.

- The slice thickness is determined by the amplitude (slope) of the z gradient as well as the bandwidth of the RF pulse (transmit bandwidth).
- If a thinner slice is desired, a higher amplitude is required. A thicker slice uses a lower amplitude gradient.
- The bandwidth of the RF pulse may also be varied to control the slice thickness. This is referred to as the *"transmit bandwidth."*
- The slice location is determined by the transmit frequencies of the RF pulse (Figure 5.15).

Frequency Encoding (Readout)

We will skip over the phase encoding gradient at this point and first examine the frequency encoding portion of the data acquisition. To sample the echo, the computer must digitally sample the signal over time (readout). During this sampling, the data points are collected and represent one "line" of data acquisition.

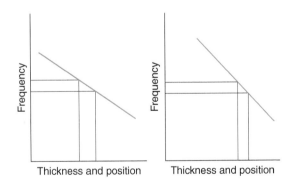

Figure 5.15 The amplitude of the slice selecting gradient (Gz) affects slice thickness. Increasing the amplitude results in a thinner slice excitation.

- If a 256-frequency encoding is selected, the system will sample the echo 256 times in the presence of the frequency encoding gradient.
- This process will produce 256 data points of data, which represent a "line" in k-space in the frequency or x direction of k-space (Figure 5.16).
- After this single sample, the computer has only enough data to reconstruct an image with a spatial resolution of 256 frequency × 1 phase.
- If we desire an image with a spatial resolution of 256 frequency × 256 phase, then we must produce 256 echoes, each distinctively encoded for the other direction (y direction) in k-space.

Phase Encoding

- The phase encoding (y) gradient is applied during the FID.
- The purpose of phase encoding is to encode spatial information into the MR signal representing a specific phase "line" in k-space.
- If a phase resolution of 256 is desired, then the pulse sequence must be repeated a minimum of 256 times;

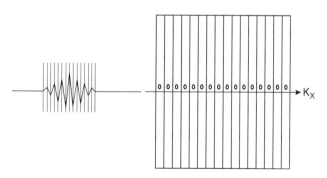

Figure 5.16 Frequency data plotted in the K_x direction.

with a different phase gradient amplitude applied each repetition.

- With each repetition, the phase encoding gradient will be applied with a different amplitude and/or polarity.
- If 256 phase encodings are prescribed by the operator, then 128 positive steps and 128 negative steps will be applied for a total of 256 steps of the phase encoding gradient (Figure 5.17).
- Some vendors refer to the phase encoding steps as *views or projections*.
- Spatial resolution may be increased in the phase direction by acquiring a greater number of phase encoding steps.
- This increases the amount of high-frequency data acquired.
- However, increasing the number of phase encoding steps increases scan time as the pulse sequence must be repeated an equivalent number of times.

In summary, k-space is a representation of the data points acquired during the MR acquisition (Figure 5.17). If 256

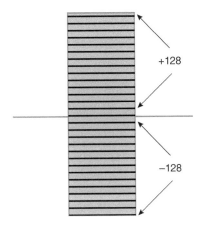

Figure 5.17 If 256-phase encodings are prescribed by the operator, then 128 positive and 128 negative steps, will be applied for a total of 256.

phase and 256 frequency encodings are desired, then 256 differently encoded echoes (phase encoding gradient steps) are acquired. Each echo is sampled 256 times during the readout period (frequency encoding). Although each data point in k-space contains information about the entire image, echoes encoded with high-amplitude phase encoding steps (either positive or negative) consist of high frequencies and contribute to spatial resolution or edge detail. These data points represent the outer edges of k-space. These data points contain little signal information and are, therefore, more noise dominant. Echoes encoded with the lower-amplitude phase encoding steps consist of low frequencies and while noise is random and occurs across all frequencies, low-frequency data (center of k-space) contribute the bulk of contrast and signal information. In fact, the "central" or low-frequency data points contribute over 95% of the resultant images contrast and signal (Figure 5.18).

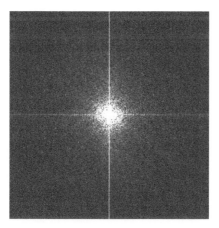

Figure 5.18 **Display of** magnetic resonance **(MR) Raw data:** data points with the greatest signal are noted in the central portion (low-frequency data), which corresponds to both the low-amplitude phase encodings (phase direction) and the central portion of the echo (frequency direction).

Number of Signal Averages

An additional parameter the MR operator must select is the number of signal averages (NSA). Some MR manufacturers refer to this parameter as the number of excitations (NEX) or number of acquisitions. NSA can easily be compared with coats of paint on a wall. If all the data points are collected twice and the signals are averaged, then the scan will be performed with two NSA, which will obviously increase the total time of the data acquisition, but does decrease the noise in the acquired voxel (resulting in an increase to the SNR).

Scan Time

Based on the previous discussion of MR data acquisition, the scan time for a 2D acquisition can be calculated as follows: $TR \times Ny \times NSA$, where TR is the pulse TR, Ny is the number of phase encodings or views, and NSA is the NSA.

The number of frequency encodings does not affect the scan time because that parameter represents the number of digital samples acquired during the brief period in which the echo forms during the readout.

Reducing Scan Time

From the beginning of routine clinical use of MRI, scientists have strived to develop ways to reduce scan time. Faster scan times are not only helpful from the standpoint of patient comfort, but they also allow for acqusition of data without the deleterious effects of physiologic motion. Many schemes are used to reduce scan times. For the purpose of this text, we will limit the descriptions to the more common techniques.

Partial Fourier

- Because of the way the data is encoded, the "upper half" of k-space is a mirror (or inverse) mathematical "image" of the "lower half."

- The right and left "halves" are a mathematical inverse.
- Partial Fourier is a technique whereby the positive or negative half of k-space is interpolated based on the values of the data in the other half.
- The top half of k-space is a product of the positive-amplitude phase encoding steps. The bottom half is a product of the negative amplitudes (Figure 5.19).
- Half Fourier takes advantage of the mathematical symmetry of k-space by acquiring slightly more than one half (either the upper or lower) and then interpolating the data for the other half, similar to the previous example.

Zero Fill

- The central (low-frequency) data in k-space, represent data acquired using the low-amplitude phase encoding steps. Recall that these data points contain most of the images' signal and therefore contrast information.
- The outermost lines (high-frequency data) contribute to the spatial resolution or edge detail.
- Zero fill is a technique that reduces scan time by reducing the amount of high-frequency data acquired.

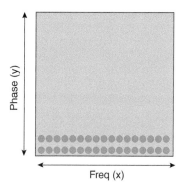

Figure 5.19 The amplitude of the phase encoding gradient effects the data points "position" in k-space along the phase or y-direction.

- For example, rather than filling all 256 lines (i.e. repeating the pulse sequence 256 times), only the middle 160 lines may be filled.
- The remaining lines of data, out to 256, are filled with zeros.
- In this example, because only the central 160 lines of k-space are acquired, an image with a spatial resolution of only 256 frequency and 160 phase can be reconstructed.
- Some manufacturers may have the operator select a matrix of 256 × 256 and then select a percentage of the matrix to be filled (e.g. 80%). In this case, only the middle 80% of k-space will be filled, and the remaining portion is filled with zeros.
- Because the outermost lines (high-frequency data) are not acquired, the scan time is reduced at the expense of spatial resolution/edge detail (Figure 5.20).

Rectangular (Fractional Phase) Field of View

Similar to zero fill, rectangular FOV results in a reduced scan time. However, this is not at the expense of spatial resolution but rather a reduction in SNR of the acquired voxel.

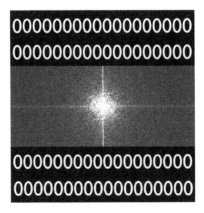

Figure 5.20 **The zero-fill technique.** Scan time is reduced by not acquiring the higher amplitude (frequency) phase views. Zeros are substituted for the magnetic resonance (MR) data. Scan time is therefore reduced at the expense of spatial resolution.

- With rectangular field of view (FOV), the number of phase encoding steps is reduced, which reduces scan time.
- Spatial resolution is maintained by reducing the FOV in the phase direction by an equivalent amount.
- The phase FOV will be reduced when the amount of change between each phase encoding step is increased.
- Spatial resolution is determined by the voxel volume, which will be discussed in detail later. The pixel size determines the in-plane resolution and is calculated by dividing the FOV (in mm) by the number of pixels in the selected acquisition matrix.
- Because the FOV in the phase direction is reduced by an amount equivalent to the reduction in phase encoding steps, the pixel size and therefore spatial resolution remain unchanged.
- The primary penalty for using a rectangular FOV technique is a reduction in signal-to-noise in the acquired voxel resulting from a reduction in the number of data points sampled.
- The reduced FOV in the phase direction may also result in aliasing in the phase FOV direction (phase wrap).
- Rectangular FOV techniques are useful when the anatomy in the phase direction is smaller than the FOV in that direction.
- As an example, rectangular FOV may be used in an axial T2-weighted acquisition of the brain (Figure 5.21). The phase FOV and the number of phase encoding steps is reduced by a factor of 0.75, resulting in a reduction of scan time without a loss of spatial resolution.

Parallel Imaging

Parallel imaging techniques use rectangular FOV as a means to reduce scan time while maintaining spatial resolution. A major difference is that parallel imaging techniques use data derived from the coil elements in a multi-coil array to reconstruct the

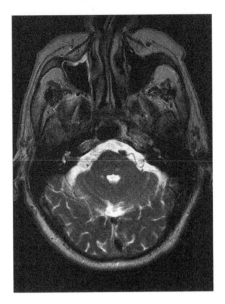

Figure 5.21 The axial sequence of the brain was acquired using a rectangular field of view (FOV). The frequency direction is anterior to posterior, and the phase direction is right to left. The FOV in the frequency direction is 240 mm and 180 mm in the phase direction. Since the phase encoding steps were reduced by the same factor (0.75), the scan time was also reduced by a factor of 0.75.

full FOV. As with the rectangular FOV technique, scan time is reduced while spatial resolution is maintained but with a reduction in SNR.

- Parallel imaging techniques require multi-channel coils.
- Scan time is reduced by means of rectangular FOV.
- A *"calibration or reference scan"* may be required prior to the acquisition of obtain data from the coil elements.
- The greater the scan time reduction, the greater the reduction in SNR (Figure 5.22).

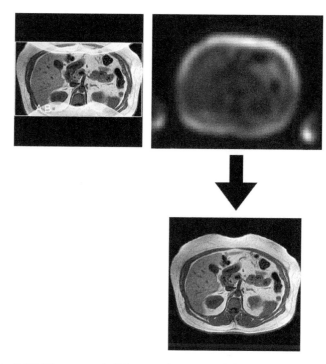

Figure 5.22 The upper left image shows an abdomen acquired with a 50% reduction in the phase FOV direction. The undersampling in the phase FOV direction resulted in the scan time being reduced by 50% but also resulted in significant aliasing. The upper right image is from the calibration or reference scan. Data from the calibration scan is used to reconstruct the full FOV, with a 50% reduction in scan time and no reduction in spatial resolution. As with rectangular FOV, the penalty is a reduction in signal-to-noise ratio (SNR).

Fast/Turbo Spin Echo

As previously discussed, the basic principles of data acquisition dictate that if an image with a spatial resolution of 256 frequency and 256 phase is desired, the pulse sequence must be repeated a minimum of 256 times (assuming a full Fourier acquisition). In this acquisition, one echo is produced and sampled during each repetition of the pulse sequence. In other words, one line of k-space is filled during each TR period. Fast spin echo (FSE) techniques (also known as RARE and turbo spin echo) fill multiple lines of k-space within a single repetition of the pulse sequence. The more lines of k-space filled in a single repetition, the shorter the overall scan time will be.

An analogy may be the writing of a book. If an author decides to write a book with 256 chapters, and each day, he or she writes one chapter, then it will take 256 days to complete the book. If three additional authors assist such that four authors are writing the book, then each day, 4 chapters will be written. In this case, it will require only 64 days to complete the book (256 ÷ 4). If eight authors are contributing to the book, then it will take only 32 days to complete the book, since eight chapters will be written each day.

- In an FSE sequence, multiple echoes will be produced within a single repetition of the pulse sequence thus filling multiple lines of k-space in a single pulse repetition.
- The number of echoes produced in a single repetition is an operator-selectable parameter known as the echo train length (ETL) or turbo factor.
- To encode each echo in a different line of k-space, a different amplitude of the phase encoding gradient is applied prior to each echo readout.
- Echoes generated following high-amplitude phase encoding gradients are encoded for the outer (high-frequency) lines of k-space.
- Echoes generated following low-amplitude phase encoding gradients are encoded for the inner or central (low-frequency) lines of k-space.
- Because the data points in the low-frequency portion of k-space are weighted more toward signal information, they will have a stronger influence on the resultant image contrast.

▪ The *effective TE* or *target TE* is the echo that is encoded for the centralmost (low-frequency) portion of k-space.
▪ The scan time for an FSE sequence is determined using the following formula:

$$\frac{TR \times \text{number of phase encodings} \times NSA}{ETL}$$

A simplified PSD shows an FSE sequence using an eight ETL (Figure 5.23). In this example, eight lines of k-space will be filled during one TR period. If 256 phase encodings were selected (256 phase lines to fill), then the pulse sequence will be repeated a minimum of 32 times, with each echo encoded for 32 lines of k-space. The effective TE will be encoded with the middle 32 phase encoding steps (i.e. ±32). Using an eight ETL, as in this example, will result in an 8x reduction in scan time.

Controlling Image Quality with FSE

Although FSE has been a tremendous tool for reducing scan times and improving image contrast at both low- and high-field strengths, it is not without caveats. The primary problem

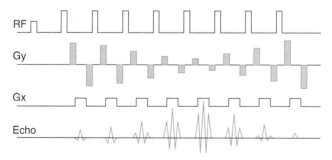

Figure 5.23 A simplified fast spin echo (FSE) pulse sequence diagram (PSD) (eight echo train length [ETL]).

is image blurring. FSE image blurring increases as the effective TE decreases and as the ETL and/or the echo spacing increases.

- Because the rate of T2 decay is exponential, there is greater change in MR signal intensity between echoes early in the train.
- Using a short effective TE, places the early echoes in the train in the central portion of k-space.
- The rapid change in signal intensities between echoes mapped to the central portion of k-space can result in image blurring.
- With a short effective TE, a short ETL is desired to minimize echo blurring.

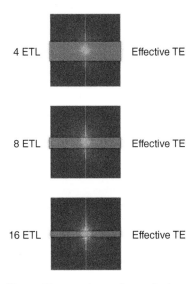

Figure 5.24 The effect of increasing echo train length (ETL) with respect to the number of lines filled by the effective time to the echo (TE). The ETL increases, the effective TE fills less of the center portion of k-space. This results in other echoes filling these "lines." Out of 256 "lines" in k-space, the middle 64 contribute over 90% of an image's contrast and signal information. Increasing the ETL results in the image's contrast becoming more of a "composite" of multiple TE times. This can lead to image blurring.

As the ETL increases, the effective TE fills less of the central portion of k-space, resulting in echoes of different signal intensities filling the central portion along with the effective TE. As in the previous statements, this factor will result in image blurring (Figure 5.24).

The echo spacing is the space or time between each echo. Increasing the echo spacing causes the ETL to extend longer over time. Because later echoes have a lower signal from T2 decay and as the signal differences between echoes increases, the result is an increase in image blurring. Some manufacturers may provide the operator direct control over the echo spacing while others may allow the operator to control the echo spacing indirectly. In this case, the receiver bandwidth is a good way to control the echo spacing. Receiver bandwidth will be discussed in more detail later. For the moment, however, increasing the receiver bandwidth will reduce the echo spacing thus reducing image blurring. Conversely, reducing the receiver bandwidth will increase the echo spacing thus increasing image blurring.

In summary, the following steps can be taken to minimize or reduce image blurring that can occur with FSE sequences:

- Increase the effective TE.
- Reduce the ETL.
- Reduce the echo spacing (increase the receiver bandwidth).

6 Magnetic Resonance Image Quality

As previously stated, Magnetic Resonance (MR) image quality is a function of contrast resolution, spatial resolution and the signal-to-noise ratio (SNR) in the acquired voxel. Having discussed image contrast, we will now examine SNR and spatial resolution. The difficulty in optimizing MR image quality is that these two characteristics often compete with each other. In most instances, when spatial resolution is increased, SNR is reduced. Increasing SNR, depending on the method chosen by the operator, can result in a reduction in spatial resolution.

Spatial Resolution

- Spatial resolution is the ability to distinguish one structure as separate and distinct from another.
- If two different structures are contained within a single voxel, they cannot be seen as two distinct structures. Their signals will be averaged in the reconstructed voxel.
- This is referred to as *"partial volume averaging."*
- Voxel volume is a determining factor in spatial resolution.
- Larger voxels result in greater partial volume averaging and therefore, reduced spatial resolution.

Rad Tech's Guide to MRI: Basic Physics, Instrumentation, and Quality Control, Second Edition. William H. Faulkner, Jr.
© 2020 John Wiley & Sons Ltd. Published 2020 by John Wiley & Sons Ltd.

- The acquired voxel is three-dimensional. The size of which is determined by the field of view (FOV) in units of millimeters (mm), the acquisition matrix (both phase and frequency), and slice thickness.
- The term *pixel* is often applied to the "face" of the voxel, which is determined by the FOV and the acquisition matrix.
- Pixel size is synonymous with the term *in-plane resolution*.
- To determine the pixel size, (1) divide the FOV (in units of mm) by the frequency matrix, (2) divide the FOV (in units of mm) by the phase matrix, and (3) multiply the answers from steps 1 and 2. The answer will be in units of millimeters square (mm^2).
- To determine the voxel volume, (1) divide the FOV (in units of mm) by the frequency matrix, (2) divide the FOV (in units of mm) by the phase matrix, and (3) multiply the answer from steps 1 by the answer from 2 and then multiply this product by the slice thickness. The answer will be in units of cubic millimeters (mm^3) (Figure 6.1).
- The FOV controls the voxel volume (as demonstrated in the previous calculation), but it is important to remember that the FOV controls the voxel volume in two dimensions.
- If the operator reduces the FOV by a factor of 2 (half), the voxel volume decreases by a factor of 4 (2^2).

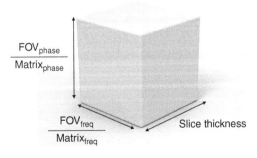

Figure 6.1 Parameters used in calculating the voxel volume.

$\dfrac{FOV_{phase}}{Matrix_{phase}}$

$\dfrac{FOV_{freq}}{Matrix_{freq}}$

Slice thickness

- Using a larger FOV and then magnifying the image for photographic purposes (making the image larger on the film) does not increase spatial resolution.
- The only way to increase spatial resolution is to reduce the voxel volume or pixel size.
- Magnification can make the image appear blurry because it magnifies the pixel.

Signal-to-Noise Ratio (SNR)

The term SNR refers to a ratio of signal in an acquired voxel to the noise in the acquired voxel. Noise is random and originates from multiple sources, including the environment, the patient, and the system's electronics. Signal comes only from the patient, or more specifically, the tissue in the voxel. To increase the SNR, the technologist must increase the signal or reduce the noise. All operator-selectable acquisition parameters affect the SNR in some way. Surface coils are also powerful tools for increasing the SNR. The following text explores the effect of various parameters on the SNR. For the purposes of this discussion, an assumption is made that all other parameters will remain unchanged. For example, when describing the effect of increasing the repetition time (TR), the assumption will be made that all other parameters will be unchanged.

Timing Parameters

- Increasing the TR increases the amount of longitudinal magnetization allowed to recover between excitation periods (TR) and will therefore result in an increase in SNR (up to a point dictated by the proton density of the tissue).
- Reducing the TR will increase the saturation of tissues and will therefore result in a reduction in the SNR.
- Increasing the time to the echo time (TE) increases the amount of transverse magnetization decay between the

excitation pulse and the sampling of the echo. The result is a reduction in the SNR.

▨ Reducing the TE reduces the amount of transverse magnetization decay between the excitation pulse and the sampling of the echo. Again, the result is an increase in the SNR.

▨ Increasing or reducing the inversion time (TI) is not as straightforward. However, if the decision is made, for example, to null the signal from fat, and the area being imaged contains a large amount of fat, then the resultant image will be a rather low SNR because the major tissue providing the signal (in this example, fat) is nulled.

▨ Selecting a TI that is slightly off the null point will result in less suppression of fat and therefore an improvement in SNR.

Flip Angle

Adjusting the flip angle of a gradient echo sequence can either increase or decrease the SNR of an image, depending on other parameters. With extremely low flip angles (e.g. 5°), the amount of transverse magnetization is rather small as is the resultant SNR. In this example, increasing the flip angle from that point will increase the SNR. There will be a point, however, when the signal will reach its maximum and will then begin to decrease as the flip angle continues to be increased. **The flip angle that produces the maximal signal for a given tissue at a given TR is known as the *Ernst angle*.**

▨ If the flip angle is below the Ernst angle, then increasing the flip angle will result in an increase in the SNR and vice versa.

▨ If the flip angle is greater than the Ernst angle, then increasing the flip angle will result in a reduction in the SNR and vice versa.

▨ The Ernst angle will be specific for various tissues and is based on the TR and the T1-relaxation time of the tissue.

Voxel Volume

As previously discussed, voxel volume controls the spatial resolution. Voxel volume also directly affects the SNR.

- Increasing the slice thickness will increase the SNR by the same amount of the change.
- Reducing the slice thickness will reduce the SNR by the same amount of the change.
- For example, if the slice thickness is increased from 3 to 6 mm, then the voxel volume will double, thus the SNR (specifically the signal) will increase by a factor of two (doubled).
- Increasing the number of phase or frequency encodings reduces voxel volume and reduces the SNR.
- Reducing the number of phase or frequency encodings increases voxel volume and increases the SNR.
- Increasing the FOV increases voxel volume and increases the SNR.
- Reducing the FOV reduces voxel volume and reduces the SNR.
- The FOV has the greatest effect on voxel volume because it affects the voxel size in two dimensions.
- For example, if the FOV is increased by a factor of 2, then the voxel volume will be increased by a factor of 4 (factor of 2 in each direction). As a result, the SNR will increase by a factor of 4.

Sampling Parameters

The term *sampling parameters* refers to parameters that control the amount of time spent sampling the acquired voxel.

These parameters include the number of signal averages (NSA), phase encodings, frequency encodings, and receiver bandwidth. Generally, when more time is spent sampling the voxel, noise decreases. However, noise is random such that, if the NSA is doubled, the SNR does not double because signal is unaffected, only noise is reduced.

Number of Signal Averages

- The NSA is somewhat analogous to coats of paint.
- For example, if an MR scan is acquired with two NSA, each line of k-space is filled twice and the signals are averaged.
- Again, because noise increases randomly, the SNR is proportional to the $\sqrt{\text{NSA}}$.
- In this example, the total scan time is twice that of a scan acquired with one NSA.
- The SNR, however, will not double, but rather, increase by $\sqrt{2}$.
- The $\sqrt{2}$ is 1.41 so increasing the SNR by a factor of $\sqrt{2}$ is the same as stating that SNR increases by a factor of 1.41.
- Increasing a number by a factor of 1.41 can also be stated as increasing by 41%.

As the relationship between SNR and NSA indicates, to double the SNR (i.e. to increase the SNR by a factor of two), the NSA will have to be increased by a factor of four ($\sqrt{4} = 2$). As mentioned, since increasing the NSA by a factor of four results in a fourfold increase in sampling time, the total scan time increases by a factor of four. Generally, attempting to increase the SNR by increasing the NSA is inefficient from the perspective of scan time (Figure 6.2).

Original NSA = 2
New NSA = 4

$$\text{New NSA} = \sqrt{\frac{\text{New NSA}}{\text{Original NSA}}}$$

$$\text{New NSA} = \sqrt{\frac{4}{2}} = \sqrt{2} = 1.41$$

Figure 6.2 Formula calculates the effects of changing the number of signal averages (NSA) on the signal-to-noise ratio (SNR).

Number of Phase Encoding and Frequency Encoding Steps

- Increasing the number of phase or frequency encoding steps also increases the number of samples taken during an acquisition.
- The SNR is proportional to $\sqrt{\text{total sampling time}}$. Therefore, increasing the number of samples by this method increases the SNR.
- An increase in the number of phase or frequency samples also reduces the voxel volume.
- The SNR is directly proportional to voxel volume. Therefore, the net effect on the SNR when the phase and/or frequency samples is increased is a reduction in the SNR.
- In other words, the effect from the reduction in voxel volume is greater than the effect from the increase in sampling time.

Receiver Bandwidth

The receiver bandwidth represents the range of frequencies sampled during the readout of the echo. Receiver bandwidth is determined by the number of frequency samples to be taken (frequency matrix) and the time required to take these samples. For example, if 256 frequency samples are collected (i.e. a 256-frequency matrix) and the readout or sampling period is 8 ms, then the receiver bandwidth will be 16 kHz (or an absolute bandwidth of 32 kHz). The relationship between the number of samples, the sampling time, and the receiver bandwidth is illustrated in Figure 6.3.

- At a field strength of 1.5 Tesla, the center frequency is $42.6\,\text{MHz/T} \times 1.5\,\text{T}$ or 63.9 MHz.
- With a receiver bandwidth of 32 kHz, the frequencies sampled will be 63.9 MHz ± 16 kHz.

$$\text{Receiver bandwidth} = \frac{\text{Frequency matrix (sample)}}{\text{Readout (sampling) time}}$$

$$32\,\text{kHz} = \frac{256}{8}$$

Figure 6.3 The relationship among the number of samples, the sampling time, and the receiver bandwidth.

▧ The frequencies sampled are "mapped" across the FOV, as illustrated in Figure 6.4.

▧ If 256 pixels are reconstructed across the frequency field of view with a receiver bandwidth of 32 kHz, then each pixel will have a value of 125 Hz (125 Hz/pixel).

▧ If one were to increase the receiver bandwidth to 64 kHz, then each pixel will have a value of 250 Hz (250 Hz/pixel).

The amount of noise in an acquired voxel depends on the range of frequencies in the acquired voxel. Therefore, if the receiver bandwidth is reduced, then the noise will be reduced, while signal is uneffected. This will result in an increase in the SNR.

▧ Reducing the receiver bandwidth reduces the noise, thereby increasing the SNR by the square root of the amount of change (Figure 6.5).

▧ The reduction in bandwidth, however, has its consequences.

▧ The FOV in the frequency direction is affected by the amplitude and duration of the readout gradient.

▧ As the receiver bandwidth is reduced, the readout gradient must increase over time to maintain the desired FOV.

▧ As a result, the minimum TE attainable will increase.

▧ Additionally, the chemical shift artifact will increase (which is discussed in detail later) (Figure 6.6).

▧ Because a chemical shift artifact is significantly less at lower field strengths, reducing the receiver bandwidth to improve the SNR is used more often on lower field strength systems.

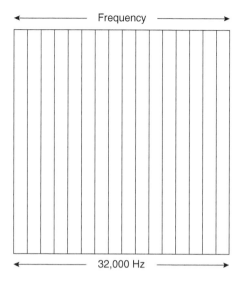

Figure 6.4 The receiver bandwidth represents the frequencies mapped across the field of view in the frequency direction.

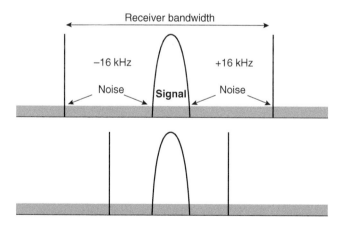

Figure 6.5 Reducing the receiver bandwidth reduces the amount of noise relative to the magnetic resonance signal.

$$32 \text{ kHz} = \frac{256}{8 \text{ msec}} \qquad 16 \text{ kHz} = \frac{256}{16 \text{ msec}}$$

Figure 6.6 The effect of receiver bandwidth on sampling time.

Surface Coils

As mentioned, the primary purpose of local (surface) coils is to improve the SNR. A smaller coil will produce a higher SNR, although less tissue is imaged (with the exception of a multi-channel coil configuration). The SNR can be optimized for a particular exam by selecting a coil that is "sized" for the anatomy being imaged.

Three-Dimensional Acquisitions

Two primary techniques are used for acquiring image data: two-dimensional Fourier transform (2DFT) and three-dimensional Fourier transform (3DTF). In actuality, classic Fourier transform is not utilized but rather Fast Fourier mathematics are utilized. Therefore, the acquisition techniques may be written as "2DFFT or 3DFFT". A 2D acquisition excites a slice of tissue selectively, and a 3D acquisition excites a slab of tissue. The "slices" in a 3DFT acquisition are reconstructed by means of additional phase encodings in the size (or z) direction. The number of slice encoding steps applied determines the number of slices reconstructed. Increasing the number of slice encoding steps through a given slab decreases the thickness of the resultant slice. For example, if a 120-mm slab were acquired with 60 phase encodings in the slice (z) direction, then the result will be 60 images, each having a slice thickness of 2 mm. If the number of slice encodings were increased to 120, then the result will be 120 images, each with a slice thickness of 1 mm (Figure 6.7).

- Scan time for a 3D acquisition is given by $TR \times Ny \times NSA \times$ the number of slice encodings (Nz).
- For this reason, the 120-partition data set previously described will have twice the acquisition time of the 60-partition data set.
- However, because SNR is proportional to the $\sqrt{\text{total sampling time}}$, the 120-partition data set will have $\sqrt{2}$ greater SNR.

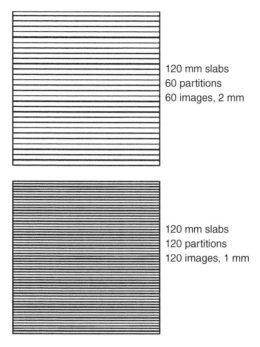

120 mm slabs
60 partitions
60 images, 2 mm

120 mm slabs
120 partitions
120 images, 1 mm

Figure 6.7 Increasing the number of slice encoding.

This property demonstrates the power of a 3D acquisition; the more slice encodings for a given slab size, the thinner the resultant slices and the higher the SNR.

Isotropic Voxels

If a 3D data set is acquired with isotropic voxels, the data set may be reformatted to produce images in any plane.

- An isotropic voxel is equal in all dimensions (i.e. a cube).
- To prescribe an isotropic data set, the operator should first select a square matrix (256 frequency and 256 phase).
- The next step is to divide the FOV, in millimeter units, by the matrix.
- The result should be selected as the slice thickness (Figure 6.8).

Matrix of 256 = 256, field of view = 280 mm
280 ÷ 256 = 1.1

1.1 mm should be selected as the slice thickness
(partition thickness)

Figure 6.8 Isotropic voxel calculation example.

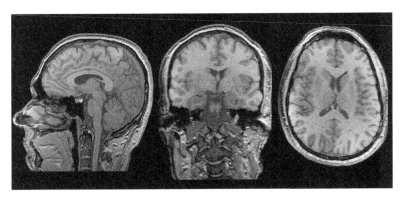

Figure 6.9 Reformatted images of a 3D sagittal acquisition.

As a practical matter, most workstations interpolate 3D data sets such that voxels need not be exactly isotropic. However, the closer to isotropic, the better the resultant image quality.

The coronal and axial images in Figure 6.9 were reformatted from a sagittally acquired 3D data set. The sagittal 3D acquisition (spoiled GRE) was acquired on a 3 T system with a slice thickness of 1 mm and a scan time of approximately four minutes.

Various scan parameters and options, including their effect on SNR, spatial resolution, and scan time, are summarized in Table 6.1.

Table 6.1 Parameter effects.

Parameter	SNR	Spatial Resolution	Scan Time
Increase repetition time (TR)	Increase	N/A	Increase
Reduce TR	Reduce	N/A	Reduce
Increase echo time (TE)	Reduce	N/A	N/A
Reduce TE	Increase	N/A	N/A
Increase receiver bandwidth	Reduce	N/A	N/A
Reduce receiver bandwidth	Increase	N/A	N/A
Increase field of view (FOV)	Increase	Reduce	N/A
Reduce FOV	Reduce	Increase	N/A
Increase slice thickness	Increase	Reduce	N/A
Reduce slice thickness	Reduce	Increase	N/A
Increase frequency matrix	Reduce	Increase	N/A
Reduce frequency matrix	Increase	Reduce	N/A
Increase number of signal averages (NSA)	Increase	N/A	Increase
Reduce NSA	Reduce	N/A	Reduce
Increase number of 3D partitions (maintain slab size)	Increase	Increase	Increase
Reduce number of 3D partitions (maintain slab size)	Reduce	Reduce	Reduce

FOV, Field of view; NSA, number signal averages; SNR, TE, echo time; TR, repetition time.

7

Artifacts

An **artifact** may be described as anything appearing on a magnetic resonance (MR) image that does not exist in the area being imaged. Technologists must learn to recognize artifacts and know what can be done to reduce or eliminate them. MR artifacts can be subdivided into several categories. The physical principles of MR contribute to the presence of artifacts. Sampling artifacts result from limitations of the techniques used to sample the MR signal. Equipment artifacts are a result of malfunctioning equipment or its failure.

Chemical Shift (Water and Fat in Different Voxels)

- As mentioned, hydrogen in fat and hydrogen in water precess at different frequencies.
- This difference in resonant frequency is referred to as chemical shift.
- Chemical shift is field-strength dependent and increases with field strength.

Rad Tech's Guide to MRI: Basic Physics, Instrumentation, and Quality Control, Second Edition. William H. Faulkner, Jr.
© 2020 John Wiley & Sons Ltd. Published 2020 by John Wiley & Sons Ltd.

- Chemical shift however, can be expressed independent of field strength as 3.5 ppm (parts per million)
- As the echo is sampled, the frequencies are "mapped" across the field of view (FOV) in the frequency direction.
- The receiver bandwidth determines the Hertz/pixel value.
- Because fat and water differ in frequency, a pixel shift occurs at fat and water interfaces.
- At 1.5 Tesla, for example, if 256 frequency encodings are selected, and if the receiver bandwidth is 32 kHz, then the frequency range within each pixel will be 125 Hz. Because the chemical shift between fat and water is approximately 224 Hz at 1.5 Tesla and assuming we have centered on the frequency of water, voxels containing fat are shifted along the frequency direction by approximately 1.8 pixels.
- Using the previous example, if the receiver bandwidth were reduced to 16 kHz, the Hertz/pixel value will be 62.5 Hz/pixel. Because the chemical shift at 1.5 Tesla is approximately 224 Hz, the pixel shift in this case will be approximately 3.6 pixels (double).
- The chemical shift artifact appears as a black or white band at fat and water interfaces and occurs along the frequency encoding direction of the FOV (see Figure 7.1).

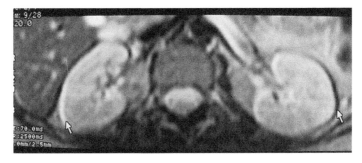

Figure 7.1 This axial acquisition through the kidneys was acquired with the frequency encoding direction along the left-to-right direction of the field of view (FOV). The chemical shift artifact is indicated by the arrows.

- Reducing the receiver bandwidth causes the chemical shift artifact to increase (greater pixel shift).
- Increasing the receiver bandwidth causes the chemical shift artifact to decrease (less pixel shift).
- A chemical shift artifact is an example of an artifact that cannot be eliminated but can only be reduced.
- As the field strength decreases, the chemical shift artifact becomes less apparent.

Chemical Shift (Water and Fat in the Same Voxel)

- Gradient echo sequences do not have the 180° radio-frequency (RF) pulse before the echo as do spin echo sequences.
- As such, gradient recalled echo (GRE) sequences do not correct for slight inhomogeneities and chemical shifts.
- At an echo time (TE) of zero (i.e. immediately following the creation of transverse magnetization) fat and water spins are in phase.
- As time passes, water spins will gain phase relative to the fat spins because of their slightly higher precessional frequency.
- Within a few milliseconds, the water spins will "catch up" to the fat spins, and once again, fat and water will be in phase.
- The timing of this cycling of the spins is field-strength dependent (as chemical shift is field-strength dependent).
- At 1.5 Tesla, fat and water spins cycle in and out of phase approximately every 2.2 msec (Figure 7.2).
- In the case of a voxel containing both fat and water, if it is sampled at a TE when the magnetic moments of the fat and water protons are 180° out of phase, the magnetic moments will cancel and result in a signal void within the voxel.

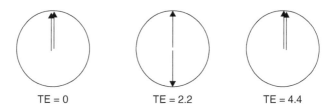

TE = 0   TE = 2.2   TE = 4.4

Figure 7.2 At 1.5 Tesla, fat and water spins cycle in and out of phase approximately every 2.2 ms.

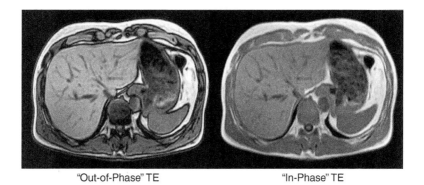

"Out-of-Phase" TE   "In-Phase" TE

Figure 7.3 The image on the left was acquired with an out-of-phase echo time (TE). The image on the right was acquired with an in-phase TE. Note the signal void in voxels which contain both fat and water (water/fat interface).

- A GRE sequence acquired when fat and water out of phase will exhibit a dark line at fat and water interfaces (Figure 7.3).
- To correct for this (i.e. to eliminate the dark line), the operator should select a TE with fat and water in phase.
- To calculate the increment of phase cycling, the following formula can be used.

$$\frac{1}{\text{Field strength}} \times 3.355$$

Example for 1.5 T

$$\frac{1}{1.5} \times 3.355 = 2.2$$

TE = 0 in phase

TE = 2.2 out of phase

TE = 4.4 in phase

Table 7.1 offers in-phase and out-of-phase TE times for various field strengths. This particular phenomenon is not observed with spin echo techniques because the 180° refocusing pulse is halfway between excitation and sampling and thus corrects for this manifestation of chemical shift.

Table 7.1 In- and Out-of-phase TE times.

Field Strength	In-Phase TE	Out-of-Phase TE	In-Phase TE
0.2 T	0	17.0	34.0
0.3 T	0	11.0	22.0
1.0 T	0	3.3	6.6
1.5 T	0	2.2	4.4

T, Tesla; *TE*, echo time.

Magnetic Susceptibility

- Magnetic susceptibility refers to the ability of a substance to become magnetized.
- Metallic objects in the body are magnetized to a greater extent compared with the surrounding tissues.
- The effect on the spins in the area of the metallic object is such that they experience a different magnetic field because of the presence of the metal.

- As a result, the spins in close proximity to the metal precess at a frequency vastly different from the spins farther away from the metal.
- The spins in the area of the metal are therefore not affected by the excitation pulse because of their frequency difference.
- The result is a signal void in the area of the metal.
- If a gradient echo sequence is used for the acquisition, this area of signal loss would be greater compared to a spin echo acquisition of the same area.
- The 180° radio-frequency (RF) pulse used in a spin echo sequence will correct for some of the inhomogeneities created by the metal. Although a signal void can still be observed in the immediate area of the metal, it will be smaller than the void produced with a gradient echo sequence.
- To further reduce the size of the signal void, fast spin echo (FSE) sequences can be used. The multiple 180° pulses used in FSE sequences further reduce magnetic susceptibility effects reducing the overall size of the signal void.
- As a clinical matter, it has long been known that GRE sequences are far superior to spin echo sequences (and to a greater extent, FSE sequences) for sensitivity to hemorrhage, particularly in the brain.
- When blood breaks down over time, hemosiderin remains, which is an intracellular storage form of iron thus producing a small local inhomogeneity.
- The 180° pulse corrects for this local inhomogeneity to the extent that it may not be visible with spin echo-based sequences.
- The presence of metal or hemorrhage is not the only source for signal loss resulting from susceptibility effects.
- In the body, tissues vary in their magnetic susceptibility.

- For example, air is hardly magnetized while tissue such as brain have a relatively high magnetization.
- When two tissues with different magnetic susceptibilities, such as air and brain matter interface, a small local gradient magnetic field is created.
- Again, spin echo-based sequences largely correct for this inhomogeneity, whereas gradient echo-based sequences do not.
- Regardless of whether spin echo or GRE sequences are used, magnetic susceptibility artifacts can be affected by several parameters.
- Magnetic susceptibility artifact is affected by field strength, voxel volume, TE and receiver bandwidth.
- As field strength decreases, magnetic susceptibility (and therefore artifact size) decreases.
- For these reasons, signal loss from magnetic susceptibility effects is less of a problem with low field strength systems.
- As voxel volume decreases, magnetic susceptibility artifact decreases.
- 3D GRE sequences that use small voxels and short TE times will also have smaller signal void artifacts from magnetic susceptibility as compared with 2D sequences that use larger voxels (and possibly longer TE times).
- As TE is reduced, magnetic susceptibility artifact is decreased.
- As the receiver bandwidth is **increased** susceptibility artifacts decrease.

Motion and Flow

Magnetic resonance imaging (MRI) uses gradient magnetic fields to encode the signals to derive spatial information. Any movement of spins can cause artifacts and/or loss of signal. The cause of motion artifacts and imaging options that may be used to reduce or eliminate them will be briefly described.

- Motion during the acquisition process is observed as a smearing or *ghosting* along the phase encoding direction.
- This effect is primarily a result of movement of spins following the application of the phase encoding gradient and the inherent time delay to the sampling or readout of the signal.
- Motion is generally not observed in the frequency encoding direction because of the usually short duration of the readout gradient and the fact that frequency encoding is performed during this readout period.
- Various techniques can be used to reduce or eliminate ghosting, depending on the type of motion or its origin.
- Motion can be subdivided into two main types: *periodic* and *aperiodic.*
- Periodic motion is characterized by motion that occurs at somewhat regular intervals.
- Examples of periodic motion include respiration, cardiac motion, blood flow, and cerebral spinal fluid (CSF) pulsation.
- Aperiodic motion is characterized by motion that occurs at irregular or random intervals.
- Examples of aperiodic motion include swallowing, peristalsis, and general body motion.
- Compensating for periodic motion is easier because the movement can be somewhat predictable and/or detectable.

Spatial Presaturation

In a spin echo sequence, flowing blood generally produces a signal void, because both the 90° and the 180° RF pulses are slice-selective. Flowing blood that receives a 90° RF pulse is not in the slice to receive the 180° pulse and thus produces no MR signal. In a multislice sequence, however, blood moves through multiple slice locations and receives multiple RF pulses. As a result, phase mismapping occurs. To reduce this artifact and produce images demonstrating signal void in vessels with flowing blood, additional RF pulses can be applied to the blood prior to it entering the imaging volume.

The term *saturation implies reduction in MR signal*. Spins are saturated when they are given insufficient time to regain longitudinal magnetization between excitation pulses. Saturated spins will produce little or no MR signal. In the case of flowing blood, a 90° RF pulse is applied outside the imaging volume (range of slices). When the blood flows into the imaging volume, it has minimal or no longitudinal magnetization as a result of the 90° presaturation pulse. When the 90° excitation pulse is applied in a slice, the blood in that slice has no longitudinal magnetization that can be directed to the transverse plane and thus no MR signal is produced.

- Spatial presaturation pulses are generally applied outside the imaging volume along the direction of blood flow.
- For example, when acquiring axial images of the neck and a hypointense signal in blood vessels is desired, presaturation pulses can be prescribed superior and inferior to the slice group.
- Because it is generally desirable to acquire spin echo sequences such that flowing blood produces no signal in the vessels, presaturation pulses are often prescribed along the direction of blood flow (typically superior and inferior).
- Using presaturation pulses with spin echo-pulse sequences provides an excellent technique for demonstrating clot and extremely slow blood flow within vessels.
- Clot and extremely slow flow will appear as hyperintense relative to fast flow from blood receiving both the 90° and 180° pulse.

Gradient Moment Nulling (Flow Compensation)

Generally, motion during an MR acquisition causes a reduction or loss of MR signal. However, it is often desirable to acquire images with bright signal from flowing blood, which can be accomplished by use of a technique known as gradient moment nulling (GMN). Other names used for this technique include flow compensation, gradient moment reduction (GMR), and motion artifact suppression technique (MAST).

- GMN, specifically first-order GMN, adds extra lobes to the frequency and slice selection gradients before sampling the echo.
- The effect is to regain phase coherence lost by moving spins, which, in turn, will produce vessels with bright signal.
- First-order GMN corrects only for constant velocity (i.e. slow, pulsatile flow) but does not correct for complex motions such as accelerated flow and jerk.
- First-order GMN only compensates for *laminar flow.*
- GMN works best when short TE times are used because it reduces the time between excitation and readout.
- GMN may also be used to reduce flow artifacts caused by CSF pulsations on T2- or T2*-weighted sequences.
- These pulsations may cause ghosting artifacts in the base of the skull on brain examinations and loss of signal in cervical spine examinations.

Compensation for Respiration

- The simplest way to compensate for respiratory motion is to eliminate it.
- Advances in hardware and software technology now make it possible to acquire sequences with such short scan times that they can be acquired during a breath-hold.

- Breath-hold sequences can now be acquired on most systems using either GRE or FSE sequences.
- In some cases, the artifact can be redirected such that the ghosting does not enter the anatomy of interest.
- For example, when imaging the cervical spine, if the phase encoding direction is anterior-to-posterior, any ghosting artifact caused by swallowing motion will be directed through the vertebral bodies and the spinal cord.
- The artifact can be redirected by swapping the direction of the phase encoding gradient to the superior-to-inferior (head-to-foot) direction. Because the artifact is originating from motion in the anterior neck, the artifact will be redirected superior-to-inferior and anterior to the area of interest.
- As an option, spatial presaturation pulses can be prescribed within the imaging FOV to remove unwanted signal.
- If the tissue is saturated, it produces little, if any, signal and thus the ghosting artifacts are reduced.

Respiratory motion artifacts are also reduced by the use of techniques known as respiratory compensation, respiratory triggering, or navigator techniques.

- Respiratory compensation, also known as ROPE (respiratory ordered phase encoding), "maps" the respiration cycles of the patient and alters the order of the phase encoding steps.
- Typically, phase encodings are applied linearly (i.e. going from maximal positive to maximal negative).
- Respiratory compensation will perform the low-amplitude phase steps (highest signal weighting, middle of k-space) during the period between breaths. The outer phase encoding steps are acquired during the period of maximal motion.
- The more evenly a patient breathes, the better the artifact suppression will be.
- With respiratory compensation, the repetition time (TR) remains as set by the operator.

▪ Respiratory triggering does not alter the order of the phase encoding steps but uses the patient's respiration cycle to trigger the scan for each TR (similar to cardiac gating).

▪ As such, the TR is dependent on the patient's respiratory rate and is not subject to a great deal of control by the operator.

▪ Navigator techniques utilize an additional RF pulse to "monitor" the movement of the diaphragm and alter the data acquisition accordingly.

▪ Spectral fat suppression techniques are sometimes used in abdominal imaging to enhance lesion conspicuity on T1- or T2-weighted sequences. A by-product of fat suppression is a reduction in respiratory ghosting artifacts resulting from the reduction of the signal from fat.

Cardiac Compensation

To produce images of the heart, it is necessary to either scan so quickly as to eliminate cardiac motion or to trigger the acquisition with the cardiac cycle.

▪ The patient first has electrocardiogram (ECG) electrodes and leads applied.

▪ The cardiac cycle is detected either by hardware built into the MR computer or by an external monitor connected to the MR computer.

▪ With some techniques, the excitation pulse for each TR is triggered by the R wave of the cardiac cycle.

▪ Each slice is excited at the same point during the cardiac cycle, greatly reducing the effects of cardiac motion.

▪ As with respiratory triggering, the TR is controlled by the patients' heart rate or the R-R interval (Figure 7.3).

▪ The QRS complex represents ventricular contraction (systole). The QRS interval, in electrocardiography, is the interval from the beginning of the Q wave to the termination of the S wave, representing the time for ventricular depolarization.

- The R wave triggers the scan.
- Scanning takes place between the R-R interval, which is now the TR (Figure 7.4).
- If the patient has a heart rate of 60 beats per minute, the scan will be triggered 60 times per minute or every second. The effective TR will therefore be 1 second or 1000 msec.
- Depending on the MR system, the operator may have to program delay times, which are played out after the R wave.
- In this case, the actual time available for imaging will be equal to the R-R interval minus any delay times.

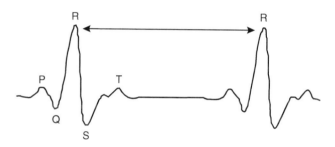

Figure 7.4 To produce images of the heart, it is necessary to either scan so fast as to eliminate cardiac motion or to trigger the acquisition with the cardiac cycle.

Cardiac gating may be used to acquire images of the heart or simply to reduce ghosting caused by cardiac motion (Figure 7.5). CSF pulsation is associated with cardiac motion. Cardiac gating may also be used to reduce CSF signal loss caused by pulsatile motion during examinations of the spine and brain.

Other types of cardiac techniques acquire data continually over multiple cardiac cycles then retrospectively sort the acquired images based on the phase of the cardiac cycle at which they were sampled.

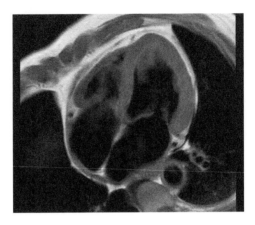

Figure 7.5 Cardiac gating may be used to acquire images of the heart or simply to reduce ghosting caused by cardiac motion.

Aperiodic Motion

Respiratory motion and cardiac motion are examples of periodic motion in that they occur at relatively consistent intervals. Aperiodic motion has no such consistency. Examples are bowel peristalsis and general patient motion.

- Bowel peristalsis can often be reduced by using anti-spasmodic drugs such as glucagon.
- Application of binding straps across the abdomen can also reduce the effects of peristalsis but may be uncomfortable for the patient or increase their anxiety about the procedure.
- Imaging the patient in the prone position is another technique that can be used to reduce the effects of peristalsis.

Patient motion can be the most frustrating problem to address. Advances in MR hardware and software technology have made it possible to acquire data in scan times of 1 minute compared with the 17 minutes it used to take. Nevertheless, if the patient is not comfortable, then movement during the examination is highly likely.

- Therefore the first step in reducing patient motion is to make the patient comfortable.
- The use of tape and restraint straps may appear to be a good idea, and in some cases, may actually be the method of choice. For patients who are able to cooperate, however, they may only serve to increase their level of anxiety about the procedure.
- Sponges can be used to support and restrain the patient without them feeling as though they are "trapped" in the magnet.
- Aperiodic and even periodic motion artifacts can also be reduced by increasing the number of signal averages (NSA).
- Sedation and even general anesthesia can be used to solve patient motion problems. However, these measures will increase the risk to the patient and require additional patient monitoring procedures and protocols to be in place.
- Rapid breath-hold techniques are now more commonly used due to improvements in hardware and software.
- Motion-reduction techniques which alter the way in which data is collected (k-space filling) are now common.
- These techniques may be known by trade names: PROPELLER, BLADE, Multi-Vane, JET, etc.
- These robust techniques can greatly reduce motion artifacts even in the case of significant patient motion (see Figure 7.6).

Aliasing

Aliasing (also known as *fold-over* or *wrap-around* artifact) occurs from tissue that is excited by the RF pulse but is outside the FOV. Aliasing is an example of a sampling artifact and occurs in both

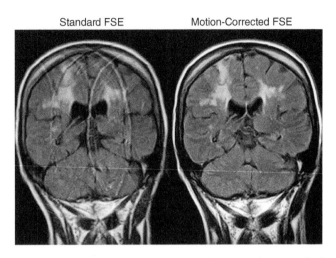

Figure 7.6 Effect of motion-correction technique when applied during a magnetic resonance (MR) examination of the brain. The standard FSE sequence is on the left and the motion-corrected fast spin echo (FSE) image is on the right.

the phase and frequency directions. Since it is easily and transparently compensated for in the frequency direction on most state-of-the-art systems, we will focus on aliasing in the phase direction.

- During data acquisition, the phase encoding gradient encodes phase shifts from $-360°$ to $+360°$ across the prescribed FOV.
- Excited tissue that falls outside the FOV has a phase shift of greater than $-360°$ and/or $+360°$ and thus has a phase value already "assigned" to a location within the FOV.
- For example, the tissue at one edge of the FOV has a phase value of $+360°$. A tissue with a phase value of $+370°$ lies just beyond the FOV.
- To the computer, the phase value of $+370°$ reads as the phase value of $+10°$ and as such, both are reconstructed and displayed in the same location.
- Essentially, this effect results in tissue from just outside the right side of the FOV to be folded over and superim-

posed over tissue inside the left side of the FOV and vice versa (assuming a right-to-left phase encoding direction).

▨ The first and simplest way to compensate for this artifact is to increase the FOV. Although this will reduce or even remove the aliased signal, it will also reduce the spatial resolution.

▨ One may also prescribe the phase encoding direction to be along the short axis of the anatomy.

▨ A specific imaging option designed to eliminate aliasing may be known as *oversampling*.

▨ An oversampling technique will increase the FOV in the phase direction and increase the number of phase encoding steps simultaneously to maintain spatial resolution.

▨ The image is reconstructed and displayed with the prescribed FOV.

▨ Although this technique will not reduce the spatial resolution, it will increase scan time.

▨ To overcome the effect on scan time, the NSA can be decreased, which can be done either manually or automatically, depending on the system software.

▨ For example, if a sequence is acquired with a 240 mm FOV, 256^2 matrix, and 4 NSA, then prescribing an oversampling technique of 100% will increase the acquired FOV to 480 mm and the phase matrix to 512. If the NSA is reduced to two, the pixel size and the scan time will remain the same. The image is reconstructed with the originally prescribed 240 mm FOV.

Gibbs and Truncation Artifact

Although two separate types of artifacts, Gibbs and truncation artifacts are both sampling artifacts that have similar appearances and both can be reduced by increasing the number of phase encoding steps.

- Truncation artifacts occur when tissues are undersampled along the phase encoding direction, and these tissues have different signal amplitudes (i.e. interfaces with high and low signal intensities, such as in a sagittal, T2-weighted sequence through the cervical spine).
- Truncation and Gibbs artifacts appear as striations or lines in the phase direction, corresponding with the high and low signal interface.
- A good example of this artifact can be observed on a sagittal cervical spine sequence with the phase encoding direction anterior-to-posterior. Truncation will appear as a line (or lines) within the spinal cord.
- On a sagittal, T1-weighted cervical spine sequence, the artifact will appear as a low signal-intensity line within the higher signal intensity of the spinal cord. On a sagittal, T2-weighted cervical spine sequence, the artifact will appear as a high signal-intensity line within the lower signal intensity of the spinal cord.
- Increasing the number of phase encoding steps will not remove the artifact; it will only make it less obvious.

Radio-Frequency Artifacts

- RF artifacts are also known as *zipper* artifacts.
- As implied, RF artifacts appear as a bright and dark band running through the image.
- These artifacts are a result of an extraneous RF signal detected by the receiver coil.
- Common causes include a leak in the RF shielding or faulty AC lighting in the scan room.
- RF leaks may come from scanning with the scan room door opened or not tightly closed.
- Leaks may also originate from electrical current coming into or originating within the scan room.

▧ Equipment such as patient monitoring devices that are not actually designed to work within an MR environment can be the cause of RF artifacts.

▧ Holes or tears in the RF shielding can result in extraneous signals entering the scan room and manifesting themselves as zipper artifacts on images.

▧ Whatever the cause, an effort should be made to locate the source of the signals and either correct or remove it.

Gradient Malfunctions

▧ Nonlinearity of gradient magnetic fields can result in images with a mild or gross distortion of normal anatomy.

▧ The cause is generally a failure of the electronics or software controlling the gradient magnetic fields.

▧ Repeated occurrences require that the system be turned over to the service engineer for service or calibration.

Image Shading

▧ Shading is described as an inhomogeneous signal across an image when using a single coil to encompass the anatomy being imaged.

▧ Shading can result from inhomogeneities in either the B_0 (static) field or the B_1 (radio-frequency) field.

▧ Shading usually requires intervention by the service engineer.

▧ Shading sometimes seen in body imaging is the result of the RF wavelength being shortened as it travels through the conductive tissues of the body. It is often referred to as the *dielectric effect* or *dielectric shading*.

▧ Dielectric shading has been greatly reduced by the introduction of new RF transmit technologies.

Inadequate System Tuning

- Nearly every MR system requires the operator to perform some type of "tuning" before scanning.
- This so-called *prescan* can include tuning the system to the resonant frequency of the patient (sometimes referred to as *center frequency*).
- Prescan tuning can also include determining the proper amount of RF energy necessary to "tip" the net magnetization 90°.
- With some systems, the receiver coil may also have to be adjusted for optimal impedance matching or loading.
- Most current systems perform these prescan tuning procedures automatically.
- However, when the automatic prescan algorithm fails or when manual tuning is not properly performed, images with inadequate quality will likely be produced.
- Symptoms can include images with severe shading, low SNR, or tissue contrasts that appear to be reversed.
- The remedy is either to properly perform the prescan tuning procedures or, in the case of a failure in the automatic prescan algorithm, have the service engineer check the system calibration.

Reconstruction Artifacts

- When the MR data are collected, they are sent to the array processor to undergo the final Fourier transform calculations.
- Because Fourier transform is a mathematical process, errors occurring during the data collection or reconstruction process have a distinctive appearance.
- Generally, reconstruction artifacts appear as geometric patterns superimposed on or across the image.

- Examples of reconstruction artifacts include the so-called *corduroy* and *herringbone* artifacts.
- Extraneous RF signals can also produce artifacts that appear similar to reconstruction artifacts.
- Whatever the cause, repeated occurrences require the attention of the service engineer.

8

Flow Imaging

Flow Patterns

Laminar flow: Friction of the blood elements against the vessel wall causes blood to flow more slowly along the walls of a vessel compared with the velocity in the center of the vessel. The result is blood flowing in smooth layers or "lamina" exhibiting a variation of flow velocities across a vessel. This produces what can be described as a parabolic shape to the flow profile. This type of flow pattern is known as *laminar flow.*

Accelerated flow: When the diameter of a blood vessel narrows, the blood spins can experience an increase in velocity, which can occur in both normal and diseased vessels and can be a source of signal loss in conventional magnetic resonance angiography (MRA) sequences.

Turbulent flow: Turbulent flow can be defined as randomly fluctuating velocities of blood flow within a vessel. Typically, turbulent flow occurs when the velocity passes a critical threshold. The presence of turbulent flow causes a signal loss in conventional MRA sequences.

Rad Tech's Guide to MRI: Basic Physics, Instrumentation, and Quality Control, Second Edition. William H. Faulkner, Jr.
© 2020 John Wiley & Sons Ltd. Published 2020 by John Wiley & Sons Ltd.

Vortex-swirling flow: Vortex flow is characterized by a somewhat circular swirling flow pattern. This type of pattern can occur immediately distal to a stenotic area and in normal vessels, particularly at bifurcations or sharp turns. The presence of vortex or swirling flow can contribute to signal loss in conventional MRA sequences.

Triphasic flow: This flow pattern is observed in normal femoral and brachial arteries. During systole, blood flows in the normal antegrade direction. During diastole, however, pressure in the vessel is reduced and the blood actually flows backward (retrograde). The flow again reverses and flows antegrade during late diastole.

Magnetic Resonance Angiography (Non Contrast)

MRA is the most common magnetic resonance imaging (MRI) application relating to imaging flow. Although the name implies that images of vessels are being produced, with conventional MRA techniques, this is simply not the case. For the most part, MRA acquires images in which the signal intensity is related to flow. The signal produced from flow (e.g. bright or dark) depends on the type of pulse sequence and imaging options selected.

Appearance of Flow in MR

Spin Echo

- The use of a spin echo pulse sequence causes normal flowing blood to appear as a signal void.
- A spin echo pulse sequence uses both 90° and 180° RF pulses.
- Both pulses are slice-selective.
- For this reason, spins of flowing blood that receive a 90° pulse are unlikely to be in the slice to receive the 180° pulse.

- To produce an MR signal in a spin echo pulse sequence, spins must "experience" both the 90° and 180° pulse.
- This effect is more prevalent when the slice is perpendicular to flow.
- MRA sequences that use spin echo-based sequences are often referred to as *black blood* techniques.

Figure 8.1 illustrates signal voids in both the left and right internal carotid and the basilar arteries (white arrows) in this patient with a large meningioma.

Gradient Echo

- A gradient echo sequence uses a gradient magnetic field to produce the echo.
- Because the gradient is not slice-selective, but rather, affects all the spins within the area of the coil, flowing blood generally appears bright.

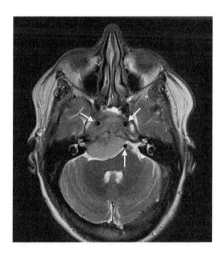

Figure 8.1 The white arrow points to the internal carotid and basilar arteries. Normal flow is seen as a signal void on spin echo sequences such as this FSE sequence.

▦ This effect is further enhanced when short echo times (TEs) are used, which minimizes the elapsed time between excitation and sampling.

▦ MRA sequences that use gradient echoes are often referred to as *bright blood* techniques.

Figure 8.2 shows nine images from a gradient echo acquisition. Note the high signal in the internal carotid and basilar arteries.

Acquisition and Display

▦ Most MRA sequences use so-called *bright blood* techniques and are acquired using gradient echo sequences (as shown in Figure 8.2).

▦ The acquisition parameters (repetition time [TR], TE, and flip angle) are selected to maximize the saturation effects

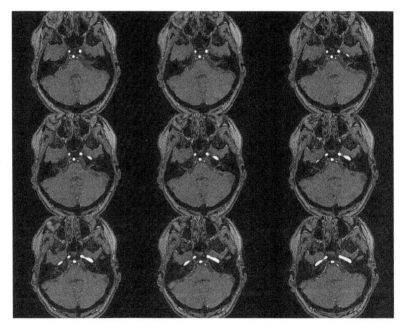

Figure 8.2 A GRE sequence.

in background tissues, thereby reducing their MR signal contribution while minimizing the saturation effects on the flowing blood.

- After the images have been acquired, they are often post-processed to produce images similar in appearance to conventional angiograms.
- The most common type of post-processing technique is *Maximum Intensity Pixel* (MIP) (Figure 8.3).
- The source images are "stacked" and the computer draws a ray through the stack at any prescribed angle. The resulting projection reveals the brightest or darkest pixel along the ray's path.
- To eliminate overlapping vessels, a sub-volume can be selected for the projections.
- One of the major advantages of MRA is the ability to produce an infinite number of projections or views from a single data set.

The MIP technique, however, has its disadvantages. Because MIP is a projection technique, there is no anatomic information. The image does not represent the vessel but rather, the signal within the vessel. In fact, MIP techniques demonstrate only the

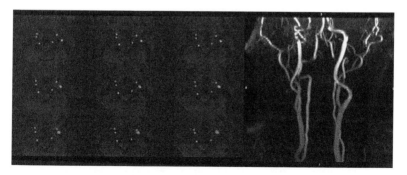

Figure 8.3 Source images from a 2D TOF acquisition and a sample Maximum intensity pixel (MIP) image.

brightest pixels. Complex flow patterns can be misrepresented as stenosis or occlusions using the MIP technique. Additionally, anything with a short T1 can appear bright on a GRE-based, time-of-flight (TOF) sequence and can appear as bright as the signal from flowing blood. Examples of these substances include fat and a hemorrhage of a specific age.

Reduction of Flow Artifacts

Two primary techniques, previously described, are used to reduce flow artifacts: gradient moment nulling (GMN or flow compensation) and spatial presaturation (*sat pulses,* sat bands). GMN is used in MRA sequences to compensate for signal loss from first-order (constant velocity) motion-flow only. Remember that GMN techniques only compensate for laminar flow. Spatial presaturation pulses can be used to remove signal from flowing blood, allowing for imaging of flow in one particular direction (e.g. superior-to-inferior or inferior-to-superior).

Signal Loss in MRA

Signal loss in MRA can occur for a number of reasons. Recognizing the origins of signal loss and optimizing the pulse sequence and its parameters are important to minimize **artifactual** signal loss.

- Flow saturation occurs when blood spins are given insufficient time to recover longitudinal magnetization between excitation pulses, which can occur in instances of slow flow or when inappropriate pulse sequence timing parameters (particularly TR and flip angle) are selected.
- Complex flow patterns (such as the patterns mentioned at the beginning of this chapter) are not easily compensated for, which often results in signal loss in an MRA sequence.

- First-order GMN (first-order flow compensation) cannot compensate for accelerated flow, turbulent flow, triphasic flow, or vortex flow.
- The amount of motion between excitation and sampling increases as the TE increases. Therefore, short TE times are important in MRA sequences.
- The chance that multidirectional flow or various velocities of flow will exist within a single voxel is increased as the voxel volume is increased.
- Additionally, magnetic susceptibility is directly proportional to both TE and voxel volume. The possibility of signal loss from magnetic susceptibility artifacts is increased as voxel volume is increased.

Two-Dimensional and Three-Dimensional Time-of-Flight

The two basic types of MRA pulse sequences are time-of-flight (TOF) and phase contrast (PC). Both sequences can be acquired as a two-dimensional (2D) or three-dimensional (3D) gradient echo acquisitions. *TOF techniques rely on flow-related enhancement to distinguish moving spins from stationary spins.*

- In 2D TOF MRA acquisitions, the images are acquired sequentially (i.e. the images are acquired and reconstructed one slice at a time).
- In this type of acquisition, the total scan time is equal to the TR × the number of phase encodings × the number of signal averages (NSA) × the number of slices.
- TR times for 2D TOF sequences are generally short (25–50 msec), and the flip angle is generally 45–70°. TE times are typically set to be as short as the hardware and/or software will allow.

- When using the TR and flip angles as described with a sequential slice acquisition, the signal from the background tissue is greatly reduced because of saturation.
- Flowing blood appears bright because unsaturated, fully magnetized blood flows into the slice replacing blood that has received RF pulses.
- The signal intensity of flow depends on blood flow velocity, the TR, and flip angle.
- For a given TR and flip angle, the higher the velocity of flowing blood, the greater the MR signal up to the point the spins are fully replaced between TR periods.
- The lower the velocity, the more RF pulses blood spins receive while in the imaging slice and thus the less intense the MR signal.
- To image slower velocities, the TR can be reduced or the flip angle can be reduced (saturation reduced).
- However, when the saturation of slower flowing spins is reduced, the surrounding tissue will be less saturated as well, which can produce less contrast between the stationary tissue and flowing bloods.
- In general, 2D TOF techniques work well for vessels with slow to moderate flow velocities.

Signal Loss with Two-Dimensional TOF

- Flow-related enhancement (FRE) is maximized when the direction of blood flow is perpendicular to the imaging slice.
- When the vessel turns and the flow is *in-plane* (i.e. parallel with the imaging slice), the spins receive additional RF pulses over time and thus experience increased saturation. This increase in saturation leads to a reduced signal from flowing spins flowing "in-plane" with the slice.

▨ Thin slices not only provide for high spatial resolution, but also improve FRE by reducing the time blood spins "spend" in an imaging slice. In most instances, 2D TOF slices range between 1.5 and 2.0 mm.

▨ Thin 2D slices require high gradient amplitudes for slice selection.

▨ Generally, the thin slices prescribed in a 2D TOF acquisition results in longer TEs and thus increases the likelihood of artifactual signal loss.

▨ Vessels can often reverse directions, causing the blood to flow back into the imaging slice, which again causes an increase in saturation of flowing spins and therefore reduction in MR signal.

▨ In the popliteal artery, the normal blood flow pattern is termed *triphasic*. Triphasic flow is characterized by the rapid acceleration of the spins as a result of the systolic contraction of the heart. The arterial blood then flows backward (superior) during diastole, followed by inferior flow.

▨ Given that triphasic flow is a complex flow pattern (i.e. not laminar), GMN (Flow Compensation will not compensate for triphasic flow resulting in a significant flow artifact.

▨ Acquiring the 2D TOF sequence with cardiac gating or triggering can greatly reduce the phase ghosting observed in the popliteal artery. However, the use of cardiac gating or triggering can often increase the overall scan time and may not be widely utilized.

▨ It is interesting to note that in the presence of a stenosis in the femoral artery, triphasic flow is not present. As such, flow artifacts are often not seen in the presence of a stenotic lesion (Figure 8.4).

Figure 8.4 demonstrates an example of an axial 2D TOF sequence through the region of the popliteal artery. The signal ghosting from normal triphasic flow is observed on

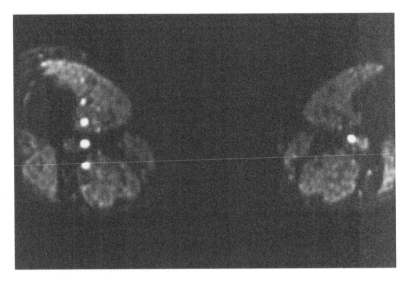

Figure 8.4 Source images of a axial 2D Time-of-Flight (TOF) acquisitionof the legs.

the patient's right side. The left popliteal artery, however, is artifact-free. In this case, the patient has a segmental occlusion on the left, resulting in a loss of the normal triphasic flow pattern.

Three-Dimensional TOF

- As the name implies, 3D TOF techniques acquire data as a 3D data set.
- The primary advantages of any 3D acquisition over a 2D acquisition are improved signal-to-noise ratio (SNR), smaller voxel volumes (improved spatial resolution), and shorter TE.
- The shorter TE and smaller voxel volumes make 3D TOF more desirable for imaging smaller vessels and less susceptible to signal loss compared with larger voxels and longer TE characteristic of 2D TOF techniques (Figure 8.5 and 8.6).

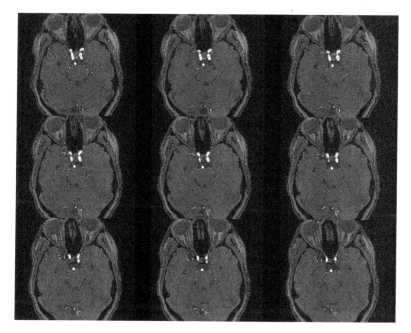

Figure 8.5 Source images from a 3D Time-of-Flight (TOF) multislab acquisition.

- The primary disadvantage to a 3D MRA acquisition is its relative insensitivity to slow flow.
- 3D TOF is the least sensitive MRA technique for imaging slow flow.
- In a 3D TOF sequence, blood flows through an imaging volume rather than a thin slice.
- As with 2D TOF, acquiring the data set such that blood flow is perpendicular to the slice direction will optimize FRE.
- However, since a volume (rather than a thin slice) of data is excited, blood spins are in the imaging volume longer and are therefore more prone to saturation.
- For this reason, lower flip angles are used with 3D TOF sequences compared with 2D TOF sequences.

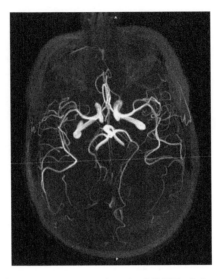

Figure 8.6 Axial Maximum intensity pixel (MIP) of the source images shown in Figure 8.5.

- In any event, 3D TOF acquisitions are less sensitive to slow flow compared with 2D TOF sequences.
- Because of the lower flip angles used in 3D TOF acquisitions, the signal from background tissue is not as suppressed compared with 2D TOF acquisitions.

Signal Loss with Three-Dimensional TOF

- The primary reason for signal loss observed in 3D TOF MRA is slow flow saturation.
- This effect can be somewhat compensated for by increasing the TR or reducing the flip angle.
- The sequence can be acquired after the intravenous administration of gadolinium, but the normal enhancement patterns of various intracranial structure often reduce the contrast between the blood flow and background tissue.

Other means of overcoming slow flow saturation include *ramped flip angle* and *multislab* acquisitions.

In a ramped flip angle acquisition, the flip angle is varied over the imaging voxel in the direction of blood flow (e.g. inferior-to-superior in an axial 3D TOF study of the circle of Willis).

For example, if the prescribed flip angle is 30°, then the flip angle in the inferior portion of the imaging slab might be 20° (30° in the middle and 40° at the top).

Multislab techniques combine the best of 2D and 3D acquisitions by acquiring multiple smaller overlapping slabs The overlapped data is discarded.

Increasing the number of slabs increases the coverage. Saturation is overcome by the use of smaller slabs.

Patient motion can present a problem. When the patient moves between slabs, misregistration can be observed in the MIP images.

Additionally, slice aliasing can result in high signal at the interface between slabs. This is often referred to as the *"Venetian Blind Artifact."*

The artifact can be reduced by increasing the amount of overlap between the slabs

PC Techniques

PC techniques rely on velocity-induced phase shifts to differentiate stationary spins from flowing spins.

A major characteristic of PC images is the complete suppression of background tissue.

Because of the way PC acquisitions are flow-encoded, they can be used to produce images that are sensitized for either slow flow or fast flow.

Depending on the type of reconstruction methods used, images indicating the direction of flow can be produced as well.

- With additional processing software, using PC to calculate flow velocities is also possible.

Flow Encoding

- Exposure to a gradient magnetic field causes spins along the axis of the gradient field to gain or lose phase, based on their position and direction of flow along the gradient.
- For stationary spins, the amount of phase gained or lost will depend on their position along the gradient, the gradient amplitude, polarity, and the amount of time the gradient field is applied.
- For flowing spins, the amount of phase gained or lost will depend not only on the gradient amplitude, polarity, and duration, but also on the velocity and direction of the flowing spins.
- In a PC acquisition, a toggled pair of bipolar gradients is used for flow encoding (Figure 8.7).
- The reconstruction "looks at" the phase shift and assigns a pixel intensity relative to the amount of phase shift.
- Stationary spins will have a zero net phase shift and thus be subtracted from the final image.
- Flowing spins, however, will have a phase accumulation and thus will be observed on the image.
- The signal intensity displayed will be based on the amount of phase accumulation, which is directly related to the velocity of the spins.
- As mentioned, the flow encoding gradients are applied as a toggled pair.
- With the second encoding, the gradient polarity is reversed.
- The two acquisitions are then subtracted to increase visualization of flow within the vessels.
- The two main methods of subtraction are complex difference and phase difference.
- Complex difference "looks at" the amount of phase shift and displays a positive pixel value of any flow with

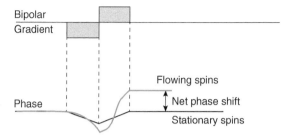

Figure 8.7 In a PC acquisition, a toggled pair of bipolar gradients is used for flow encoding.

a velocity greater than zero. The complex difference subtraction method is commonly used with thick slab acquisitions.

- Phase difference "looks at" the angle (ϕ) between the two-phase shifts produced by the toggled gradient pair and displays flow direction by pixel signal (black or white).

Velocity Encoding

- The operator can select the velocity sensitivity of a PC acquisition. That is, the operator can choose to make the flow encoding sensitive to slow or fast flow velocities (Figure 8.8).
- The parameter is referred to as the *velocity encoding* (VENC).
- VENC determines the amplitude and duration of the flow encoding gradients.
- Low values of VENC highlight slower flow and use stronger flow encoding gradients.
- High values of VENC highlight faster flow and use weaker flow encoding gradients.
- For example, if a VENC of 40 cm/sec is selected, then the flow encoding gradients will be applied such that spins

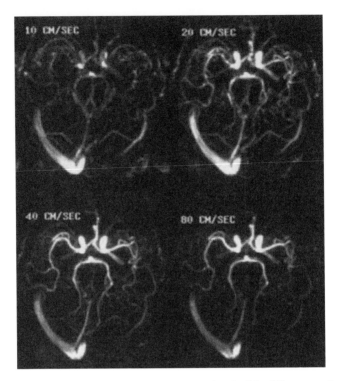

Figure 8.8 Example of PC sequences acquired with different velocity encoding (VENC) values. Note the lower VENC (upper left) shows more venous (slower) flow while the higher VENC value (lower right) shows the faster arterial flow.

flowing at 40 cm/sec will experience maximal phase shift (180°).

- With the complex difference subtraction, the reconstruction technique cannot differentiate between spins flowing faster than the VENC value and the spins flowing slower than the VENC value. Both values will be reconstructed with lower signal.

- When using phase difference subtraction, spins flowing faster than the VENC value have phase shifts of spins flowing in the opposite direction and are displayed as such.

▨ These reconstruction errors are known as aliasing.

▨ One way to consider the VENC is to say that it represents the fastest velocity that can be displayed without aliasing.

In summary, the major advantages of PC include:

▨ Complete suppression of background (nonflowing) spins.

▨ The ability to image slow or fast flow.

▨ The ability to acquire information relating to flow direction.

▨ The ability to calculate flow velocity.

Contrast Enhanced MRA (CE-MRA)

CE-MRA techniques are acquired following the fairly rapid injection of a gadolinium-based contrast agent (GBCA). CE-MRA techniques largely eliminate flow artifacts seen with TOF and PC techniques. The image contrast is based on T1-relaxation time differences between the gadolinium "enhanced" blood and the saturated background tissues (Figure 8.9).

▨ A rapid 3D spoiled gradient echo technique is used for the acquisition.

▨ It is most often acquired as a coronal acquisition.

▨ The GBCA agent is injected at rate of 1.0–2.0 ml/sec.

▨ The GBCA "bolus" is immediately followed by a saline flush.

▨ Typically, no less than 20 ml of saline is utilized and it is injected at the same rate as the GBCA.

▨ The main purpose of the saline flush is to keep the GBCA in a relatively "tight" bolus and assist in moving it through the vascular system to the vessels of interest.

▨ The dose and/or volume of the GBCA depends on several factors, however, as with any administration of a GBCA,

(a) (b) (c)

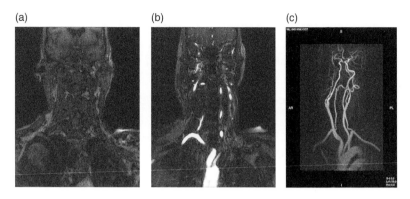

Figure 8.9 Images show the rapid 3D spoiled gradient echo prior to the injection of the gadolinium-based contrast agent (GBCA), the 3D data set acquired when the GBCA is at maximum concentration in the carotid arteries and the resultant Maximum intensity pixel (MIP) projection.

the decision to administer a GBCA, the specific agent to be used and the dose is the responsibility of the radiologist supervising the examination.

- The most common type of GBCAs utilized for CE-MRA exams are classified as *"Extra-cellular Fluid Space (ECF) Agents."*
- Following the injection of an ECF agent, the agent rapidly disperses to the extra-cellular fluid space.
- The GBCA is therefore only at maximum concentration in the vessels of interest for a few seconds.
- It is, therefore, vital that the acquisition be timed so that the low-frequency data (center of k-space) is acquired when the GBCA is at maximum concentration in the vessels of interest.
- For a CE-MRA acquisition, the low-frequency data (center of k-space) is acquired first.
- The techniques for filling k-space in this manner may be referred to as: "Centric," "Elliptical," "Elliptic" or something similar.

- Given that the low-frequency data is to be acquired in the few seconds that the GBCA is at maximum concentration, timing techniques are utilized to ensure accuracy in timing the start of the acquisition.
- The technique utilized will depend on system capabilities and vendor preference. However, common timing techniques include: *Real-time Imaging ("Bolus Track," "CareBolus"), Test Bolus and Automated Bolus Detection (i.e. "Smart Prep").*

9 Diffusion and Perfusion Imaging

Diffusion-Weighted Imaging (DWI)

Diffusion refers to the motion of extracellular fluid. A DWI therefore is one where the image contrast is based on the amount of extracellular fluid motion. The amount of diffusion is expressed by a tissue's *"Apparent Diffusion Coefficient (ADC)."* In the presence of cellular swelling (edema), diffusion, and therefore, the ADC is reduced. Many types of pathology result in a reduction in the ADC of tissues.

In order to detect subtle differences in the amount of extracellular fluid motion, the acquisition must be made sensitive to motion on the order of 5–12 μm per TR cycle. Therefore, it is critical that the effect of bulk patient motion be minimized. To accomplish this, the most common type of pulse sequence utilized for DWI is *"Echo Planar Imaging"* (EPI). An EPI sequence produces a train of gradient echoes by rapidly oscillating the readout gradient. The phase gradient is "blipped" between each oscillation of the readout gradient so that each echo fills a separate line of k-space (Figure 9.1).

Rad Tech's Guide to MRI: Basic Physics, Instrumentation, and Quality Control, Second Edition. William H. Faulkner, Jr.
© 2020 John Wiley & Sons Ltd. Published 2020 by John Wiley & Sons Ltd.

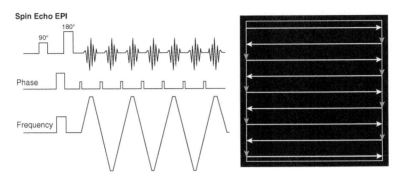

Figure 9.1 A pulse sequence diagram of a spin echo EPI (SE EPI) pulse sequence (Lt). K-space filling with a single-shot EPI sequence (Rt).

Echo Planar Imaging (EPI)

- Filling all of k-space in a single TR period of an EPI acquisition is referred to as *"Single-Shot EPI."*
- There are two main types of EPI sequences: Spin Echo EPI (SE EPI) and Gradient Echo EPI (GRE EPI).
- The name refers to the "root" or "excitation" part of the pulse sequence. With either sequence, the echoes are produced by the oscillation of the readout gradient (Figure 9.2).
- Generally, SE EPI is used for DWI and GRE EPI is used for Perfusion-Weighted Imaging (PWI) and so-called "functional MRI or fMRI" exams.
- EPI is considered one of the most rapid data acquisition techniques.

Diffusion-Weighted Imaging (DWI)

- For DWI imaging, a T2-weighted SE EPI sequence is utilized.
- To add diffusion-weighting to the image, two additional gradient pulses are added prior to and after the 180° pulse in the SE EPI sequence.

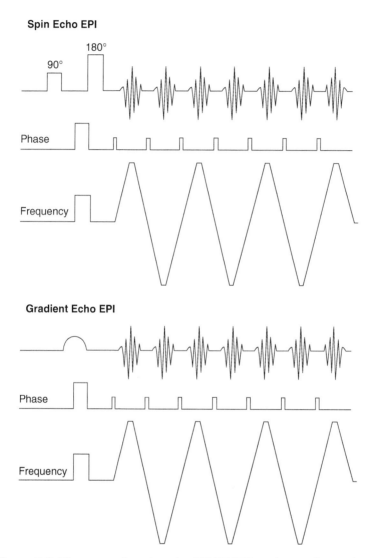

Figure 9.2 Diagrams of a spin echo EPI (SE EPI) and a gradient echo EPI (GRE EPI) sequences.

- The amplitude, duration and time between the gradient applications is given by an operator-selectable parameter known as the *"b-value."*

- With no diffusion gradient application, the image is said to be acquired with a b-value of 0 (zero).

- **Increasing the b-value, increases diffusion-weighting** (Figure 9.3).

- Diffusion can only be measured in one direction at a time. For this reason, the sequence is acquired first with no diffusion gradient applied (b-value = 0) then with the diffusion gradient applied in each direction (slice, phase, readout).

- The diffusion data from each direction is then averaged to produce the *"Isotropic Diffusion-Weighted Image."*

- **Restricted diffusion will appear hyperintense (bright) on the Isotropic DWI.**

- Although with a b-value of 1000 (for example) the image has considerable diffusion-weighting, the image still has contrast based on T2.

- Because of the T2 contribution to the image contrast, it may not be possible to determine if increased signal seen on the isotropic DWI is due to restricted diffusion or an increase in the tissue's T2-relaxation time.

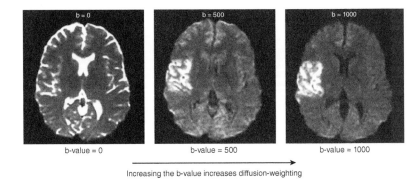

b-value = 0   b-value = 500   b-value = 1000

Increasing the b-value increases diffusion-weighting

Figure 9.3 Increasing the b-value increases diffusion weighting.

- This increase in signal due to T2 contrast is referred to as *"T2 shine-through."*
- In order to remove the effects from T2 shine-through, an *ADC map* or *image* can be produced.
- On an ADC image, restricted diffusion will appear hypointense (dark), while T2-effects will appear hyperintense (bright) (Figure 9.4).

Perfusion-Weighted Imaging (PWI)

With current technology, it is possible to obtain PWIs without having to administer a gadolinium-based contrast agent (GBCA). Those techniques may be referred to as "Arterial Spin Labeling" or something similar. For the purposes of this text, only the technique which requires the administration of a GBCA will be discussed.

GBCAs shorten both T1- and T2-relaxation times of water-based hydrogen protons. When administered at standard dose and concentration, T1-effects dominate. However, when administered at higher doses and/or when a higher concentration is present in the vessels and/or tissues, T2-shortening effects dominate.

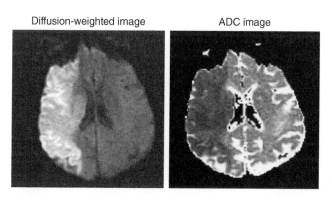

Diffusion-weighted image   ADC image

Figure 9.4 Diffusion-weighted imaging (DWI) apparent diffusion coefficient (ADC) images in a patient with stroke. Note that the stroke is hyperintense on the DWI exam and hypointense on the ADC image.

This results in a decrease in the T2- and, more significantly the T2*-relaxation times of tissues. The images in Figure 9.5 demonstrate the reduction in signal on images acquired with a GRE EPI due to the T2*-shortening effects of the GBCA bolus.

- When using a GBCA for PWI, the acquisition technique may be referred to as "Dynamic Susceptibility-Weighted Imaging."
- The pulse sequence is either a 2D or 3D gradient echo EPI sequence.
- The entire brain should be imaged every one to two seconds.
- The imaging begins first. After a short delay (six to eight seconds), a standard dose of GBCA is delivered at a rate of preferably 4–5 ml/s. This is followed by a 20 ml bolus of saline delivered at the same injection rate.
- As the GBCA flows through the vascular system in a concentrated bolus fashion, the T2*-relaxation time of the

Gradient Echo EPI w/TE of 60 msec

Prior to bolus arrival   At bolus peak

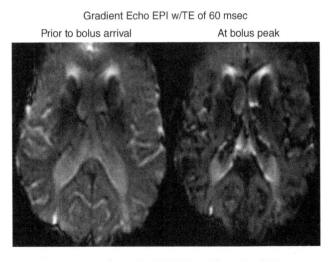

Figure 9.5 A gradient echo EPI (GRE EPI) with a TE of 60 msec prior to the arrival of the bolus of a GBCA (left) and at the time of bolus peak (right).

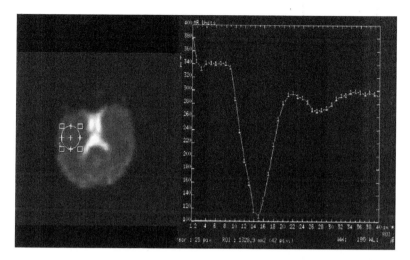

Figure 9.6 Demonstrates normal perfusion. Notice that because of the T2* shortening effects of the gadolinium-based contrast agent (GBCA) bolus, signal drops and the GBCA flows into the brain.

surrounding tissues is shortened, resulting in a *drop in signal* (see Figure 9.6).

- Using a GRE EPI, the administration of a GBCA in a bolus as described above, can decrease the T2* of tissues by 50–80%.
- For an active tumor, the amount of blood flow in the tumor area will likely be increased and the tissue is said to be *hyper-perfused.*
- In the case of an ischemic stroke, the blood flow will either be decreased or exhibit late arrival to the area of the stroke and the tissue is said to be *hypo-perfused.*

DWI and PWI in a Hyperacute Stroke

- When imaging a stroke in the hyperacute phase (first six hours), a diffusion defect (restricted diffusion) may or may not be seen.
- Perfusion imaging is necessary to fully assess a hyper-acute stroke.

78 y.o. female 3 hours after acute onset of aphasia
during cardiac catheterization

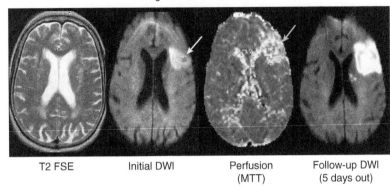

| T2 FSE | Initial DWI | Perfusion (MTT) | Follow-up DWI (5 days out) |

Figure 9.7 Three hours after the onset of acute aphasia, the T2-weighted FSE sequence does not show the hyperacute stroke. The isotropic diffusion-weighted image (DWI) shows an area of restricted diffusion. The perfusion-weighted image (PWI) shows a larger area of abnormal perfusion (increased transit time). Due to underlying medical issues and available treatment options at that particular time, the patient was not a candidate for treatment. Note that five days later, the size of the diffusion defect has grown to match the size of the perfusion defect.

▨ Any difference between a diffusion abnormality and a perfusion abnormality is referred to as the penumbra and often represents "treatable brain" if perfusion can be restored in a timely manner (Figure 9.7).

10 Gadolinium-Based Contrast Agents

Characteristics, Composition and Structure

- Gadolinium ($_{64}$Gd) is a rare earth metal in the lanthanide series of elements.
- It has seven (7) un-paired electrons and as such, is paramagnetic.
- Gadolinium, like other heavy metals is toxic in its pure form.
- For Gadolinium-Based Contrast Agents (GBCAs), the gadolinium is bound to an organic chemical called a "ligand."
- An example of a ligand used in GBCA is diethylenetri-aminepentaacetic (DTPA).
- When a metal atom is bound to a ligand, the molecule is referred to as a *"Chelate."*
- The purpose of administering gadolinium as a chelate is so that it can be removed from the body by glomerular filtration.

Rad Tech's Guide to MRI: Basic Physics, Instrumentation, and Quality Control, Second Edition. William H. Faulkner, Jr.
© 2020 John Wiley & Sons Ltd. Published 2020 by John Wiley & Sons Ltd.

- There are two types of GBCA chelate structures: Linear and Macrocyclic.
- In general, a macrocyclic chelate has a stronger bond to the gadolinium ion vs. linear chelates. However, differences in stability within each class of agent exist.

Effect on Water Protons' Relaxation Times

- The majority of the GBCAs in use today are classified as *"Extracellular Fluid Space Agents" (ECF agents)*.
- Water is a very small molecule (~ 3 Å) and, therefore, has a very rapid molecular tumbling rate. As such, water protons have a long T1- and T2-relaxation time.
- As previously mentioned, gadolinium is paramagnetic.
- The GBCA molecule is much larger than a water molecule and therefore it has a much slower molecular tumbling rate.
- When a GBCA molecule gets within approximately 3 Å of a water molecule, the molecular tumbling rate of the water slows.
- This results in a shortening of both the T1- and T2-relaxation times of the water-based hydrogen protons.
- In normal doses and concentrations, the T1-effects dominate.
- In higher doses and concentrations in the tissues, the T2-effects dominate (see Perfusion-Weighted Imaging in Chapter 9).
- The amount of change in the relaxation times of water-based protons is given by the relaxivity of the contrast agent.
- Some agents, due to their chemical composition, exhibit either protein interaction or protein binding.
- This interaction and/or binding with proteins results in an increase in relaxivity (effectiveness for a given dose).
- A common imaging option to use when acquiring T1-weighted images following the administration of a GBCA is spectral fat saturation.

GBCA Dose and Safety

- The standard dose for **all** Extracellular Fluid Space (ECF) agents in clinical use today is 0.1 mmol/kg.
- The amount administered in milliliters (ml) depends on the molar concentration of the agent.
- To calculate the volume to be administered, the patient's weight (in kg) is multiplied by the dose (0.1). The product is then divided by the molar concentration (see Figure 10.1).
- Acute adverse events following the injection of a GBCA have the same classification and treatment as acute adverse events following the injection of an iodinated contrast agent.
- Acute adverse event rates for **all** GBCAs are well below 5%.
- **Currently**, the only known chronic adverse reaction observed in some patients following the administration of some (but not all) GBCAs is *Nephrogenic Systemic Fibrosis (***NSF***)*.

Determining Volume for Standard Dose

Dose is determined by the **amount of gadolinium** not the volume of the agent administered

Standard Dose: 0.1 mmol/kg

80 kg patient

0.5 molar concentration agent	1.0 molar concentration agent
$80 \times 0.1 / 0.5 = 16$ ml	$80 \times 0.1 / 1.0 = 8$ ml
	Lower volume same dose

Figure 10.1 Calculation for volume to be administered based on the molar concentration of the gadolinium-based contrast agent.

- Given that the gadolinium chelates are excreted via the kidneys, GBCAs will remain in the body longer in patients with reduced renal function.
- In many instances, a patient's renal function may be assessed prior to the administration of a GBCA.
- The most commonly used metric for renal function (with regard to MRI) is *"Estimated Glomerular Filtration Rate (eGFR)"*.
- The American College of Radiology (**ACR**) classifies the agents based on their risk of NSF.
- Group I agents are those with the most documented cases of NSF and are contraindicated (contained in the package labeling) in patients with an eGFR <30 ml/min.
- Group II and III agents have no such contraindication although **all** agents currently have a labeled warning regarding NSF.
- The use of any GBCA for a purpose not contained in the package labeling is referred to as *"off-label"* use.

Index

Rad Tech's Guide to MRI: Basic Physics, Instrumentation,
and Quality Control, Second Edition. William H. Faulkner, Jr.
© 2020 John Wiley & Sons Ltd. Published 2020 by John Wiley & Sons Ltd.